DENTAL ASSISTANTS
AND HYGIENISTS

DENTAL ASSISTANTS AND HYGIENISTS

A Practical Career Guide

KEZIA ENDSLEY

ROWMAN & LITTLEFIELD
Lanham • Boulder • New York • London

Published by Rowman & Littlefield
An imprint of The Rowman & Littlefield Publishing Group, Inc.
4501 Forbes Boulevard, Suite 200, Lanham, Maryland 20706
www.rowman.com

6 Tinworth Street, London, SE11 5AL, United Kingdom

British Library Cataloguing in Publication Information Available

Library of Congress Cataloging-in-Publication Data

Names: Endsley, Kezia, 1968– author.
Title: Dental assistants and hygienists : a practical career guide / Kezia Endsley.
Description: Lanham : Rowman & Littlefield, 2019. | Series: Practical career
   guide | Includes bibliographical references.
Identifiers: LCCN 2018042079 (print) | LCCN 2018043179 (ebook) |
   ISBN 9781538111826 (Electronic) | ISBN 9781538111819 (pbk. : alk. paper)
Subjects: LCSH: Dental assistants—Vocational guidance. | Dental hygienists—
   Vocational guidance.
Classification: LCC RK60.5 (ebook) | LCC RK60.5 .E53 2019 (print) |
   DDC 617.6/0233—dc23
LC record available at https://lccn.loc.gov/2018042079

♾️™ The paper used in this publication meets the minimum requirements of American
National Standard for Information Sciences—Permanence of Paper for Printed Library
Materials, ANSI/NISO Z39.48-1992.

Printed in the United States of America

To Christopher,
who makes me so proud

Contents

Introduction

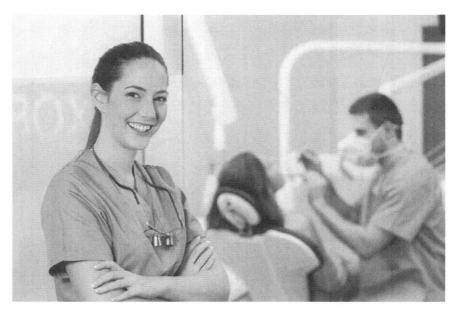

A career in dental health can be lucrative and fulfilling.

Careers in Dental Health

Welcome to careers in dental and oral health! If you are interested in a career in the dental health field, you've come to the right book. These are the professions traditionally called dental assistants and dental hygienists (also called oral hygienists). They assist and complement the work that the dentist and the entire dental team do. Dental hygienists provide services such as teeth cleaning, examination of teeth and gums for signs of decay and disease, and other preventive and maintenance oral care. Dental assistants also provide patient care, including giving X-rays and perhaps even performing scheduling and record-keeping tasks.

There is a lot of good news about this field and it's a smart career choice for anyone with a passion to help people improve their dental health and enjoy working with others. It's a great career for people who get energy from working with other people and work well in a team setting. Job demand is high and job outlook for the next decade is much better than the average profession.

When considering any career, your goal should be to find your specific nexus of interest, passion, and job demand. Yes, it is important to consider job outlook and demand, educational requirements, and other such practical matters, but remember that you'll be spending a large portion of your life at whatever career you choose, so you should also find something that you enjoy doing and are passionate about. Of course, it can make the road easier to walk if you choose something that's in demand and lucrative.

A CAREER IN DENTAL HEALTH

This book covers in detail three main areas of dental health that have proven to be stable, lucrative, and growing professions. These are:

- Dental assistants
- Dental hygienists
- Dental technicians

Be sure to check out the Bureau of Labor Statistics website at https://www.bls.gov/ooh/healthcare/home.htm for current US information about these professions and related healthcare professions.

So what exactly do these people do on the job, day in and day out? What kind of skills and educational background do you need to succeed in these fields? How much can you expect to make, and what are the pros and cons of these various fields? Do these career paths have a bright future? Is this even the right career path for you? How do you avoid burnout and deal with stress? This book can help you answer these questions and more.

"Talking to patients about good cleaning, about how to take care of their mouths, about how disease in your mouth can affect your entire body, are important parts of the job. In fact, educating patients about good oral health is a very large part of the job."—Catherine Kimmey, dental hygienist

For these professions, the book covers the pros and cons, the educational requirements, projected annual wages, personality traits that match, working conditions and expectations, and more. You'll even read some interviews from real professionals working in these industries. The goal is for you to learn enough about these professions to give you a clear view as to which one, if any, is a good fit for you. And, if you still have more questions, we will also point you to resources where you can learn even more.

An important note. Regardless of the career you might choose, to succeed in any medical and healthcare profession, you need to have a lifelong curiosity and love of learning. Your education won't be over once you finish your degree. In fact, maintaining current on certifications and meeting or exceeding continuing education requirements (usually set forth by some governing board and/or by state regulations where you practice) is all very important in healthcare careers such as these.

THE MARKET TODAY

The good news is that the United States Bureau of Labor Statistics forecasts that healthcare in general will be the fastest growing field between the decade of 2016 and 2026 (see https://www.bls.gov/emp/ for a full list of employment projections). This includes the dental health professions. Not only does this translate into job security, but it also means that more new positions are being created within the healthcare industries every year.

The demand for jobs in dental care continue to grow in the United States due to several factors:

- We have a large elderly population, as the generation of "baby boomers" continues to age. This elderly population needs more frequent dental intervention and care. In fact, the success of preventive dentistry means that the older population is keeping their teeth longer and will be needing more regular dental care.
- Ongoing studies and research have shown a link between oral health and general health (including cardiovascular health), which is increasing the demand for preventive dental services.
- Treatments in the dental profession continue to evolve and be more complicated, requiring skilled professionals.

- With the focus on preventive care, dentists need to employ more dental hygienists than ever to meet the increased demand for dental services.

Chapter 1 covers lots more about the job prospects of these professions and breaks down the numbers for each one into more detail.

What Does This Book Cover?

The goal of this book is to cover all aspects of your search for a dental healthcare degree and explain how the professions work and how you can excel in them. Here's a breakdown of the chapters:

- Chapter 1 explains the different careers in the dental health umbrella covered in this book. You'll learn about what people in these professions do in their day-to-day work, the environments where you can find these people working, some pros and cons about each career path, the average salaries of these jobs, and the outlook in the future for all these careers.
- Chapter 2 explains in detail the educational requirements of these different fields, from bachelor's degrees to certificates after high school. You will learn how to go about getting experience (in the form of shadowing, internships, and fieldwork) in these fields before you enter college as well as during your college years. You'll also learn about the certifications, licensing, and registrations you need (usually set forth by a governing board and/or by state regulations where you practice) in order to practice safely and legally.
- Chapter 3 explains all the aspects of college and postsecondary schooling that you'll want to consider as you move forward. You will learn about the great schools out there and how to get the best education for the best deal. You will also learn a little about scholarships and financial aid and how the SAT and ACT tests work.
- Chapter 4 covers all aspects of the interviewing and résumé-writing processes, including writing a stellar résumé and cover letter, interviewing to your best potential, dressing for the part, how to communicate effectively and efficiently, and more.

Where Do You Start?

You can approach the dental health field in several different ways—whether you start immediately after high school or pursue a college degree first—depending on your long-term goals and interests. Are you more interested in finding a stable and in-demand position right after high school, or would you rather pursue an associate's degree and begin working directly with patients as a result? Are you a technical-minded person who would enjoy working in a lab setting behind the scenes, or do you feel that you would be great at working with and helping people? Are you comfortable taking clinical and written board examinations, or is your strength a hands-on approach? Are you better with kids and babies, or do you enjoy working with the elderly?

The good news is that you don't need to know the answers to these questions yet. In order to find the best fit for yourself in the dental health professions, you need to understand how these jobs work. That's where you'll start in chapter 1.

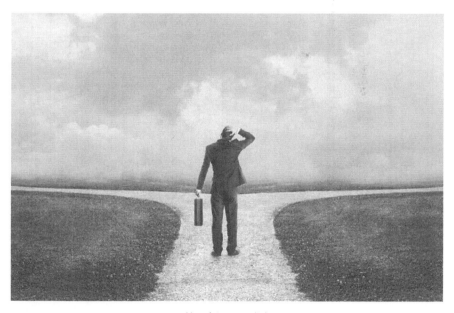

Your future awaits!

Why Choose a Career in the Dental Health Field?

You learned in the introduction that the dental health field, which includes dental assistants, dental hygienists, and dental technicians, is large, healthy, and growing. You also learned a little bit about how it's different from a career in dentistry or medicine, yet related. You also were reminded that it's important to pursue a career that you enjoy, are good at, and are passionate about. You will spend a lot of your life working; it makes sense to find something you enjoy doing. Of course, you want to make money and support yourself while doing it. If you love the idea of helping people for a living, you've come to the right book.

In this chapter, we break out these professions and cover the basics of each. The nice thing is that no matter what degree of postsecondary education you can/want to pursue, there is a way for you work in the dental health field. After reading this chapter, you should have a good understanding of each of these careers and can start to determine if one of them is a good fit for you. Let's start with the dental assistant.

What Is a Dental Assistant?

Dental assistants work in many different dental settings and help the dentists they work with provide excellent dental care in the most efficient way possible. They are valuable members of the dental care team. Depending on the type of office you work in (orthodontic, pediatric dentistry, periodontics, and even veterinary), your job will bring special challenges and rewards. The best dental assistants have excellent communication skills and enjoy working with others.

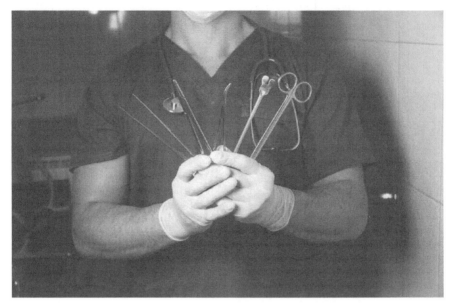

Dental assistants provide help to the dental team in numerous ways.

The dental assistant job is among the most diverse in the dental office. Dental assistants perform many tasks that require interpersonal and technical skills. States do have different regulations, so the duties and tasks that dental assistants perform will depend on where you practice. However, responsibilities often include the following:[1]

- Helping dentists during treatment procedures
- Taking and developing dental X-rays
- Recording patient medical history and taking blood pressure and pulse
- Developing infection control protocols and preparing and sterilizing instruments and equipment
- Helping patients feel comfortable before, during, and after dental treatments
- Providing patients with guidelines for oral care after surgery or other dental treatment procedures
- Teaching patients good oral hygiene techniques to maintain dental health (toothbrushing and flossing)
- Taking impressions of patients' teeth for casts

- Performing office management tasks
- Communicating with patients and suppliers (scheduling appointments, answering the telephone, and billing and ordering supplies)

In addition to good interpersonal skills, dental assistants need to have manual dexterity and be organized and reliable. The types of settings that dental assistants often work in include:

- General dental practices (single-doctor and group settings)
- Specialty practices, such as oral and maxillofacial surgery (removal of teeth and correction of facial deformities), orthodontics and dentofacial orthopedics (straightening teeth with braces or other appliances), endodontics (root canal treatment), periodontics (treatment of gum problems), prosthodontics (replacement of lost teeth), and pediatric dentistry (treatment of children)
- Public health dentistry, including settings such as schools and clinics
- Hospital dental clinics, assisting dentists in the treatment of bedridden patients
- Dental school clinics, assisting dental students as they learn to perform dental procedures

If you become "burned out" working directly with patients, you still have different opportunities as a dental assistant. You could, for example, process dental insurance claims at an insurance company, work at a vocational school or community college teaching others to be dental assistants (which may require associate or baccalaureate college degrees), or become a dental product sales representative.

Postsecondary education (usually a certificate or diploma or even an associate's degree) is a sure-fire way to find employment, but you can begin a career in dental health without college-level courses through on-the-job training in a dental office or through high school work-study programs. At this time, there are about 270 American Dental Association (ADA)–accredited dental assisting education programs in community and technical colleges in the United States, which are a minimum of one academic year in length.[2] Visit the ADA website's listing of accredited programs to find a good one close to you (see www.ada.org/en/coda/find-a-program).

Chapters 2 and 3 cover the educational and professional certification requirements in more detail.

INTERESTING DENTAL-RELATED FACTS[3]

- Dentistry is one of the oldest medical professions. Hesy-Re was an Egyptian scribe who lived around 2600 B.C. and is recognized as the first dental practitioner.
- Paul Revere, American Patriot known for warning the Colonial troops that the British were coming, was also trained as a dentist.
- Edward H. Angle started the first school of orthodontics in 1901 and created a simple classification for crooked teeth in the late 1800s that is still used today.
- The first dental X-ray was used in 1896.
- The first university-affiliated dental institution, the Harvard University Dental School, was founded in 1867.
- By 1873, the Colgate company had mass produced the first toothpaste. Mass-produced toothbrushes followed a few years later.
- The first African American to earn a dental degree dates all the way back to 1869.
- Americans did not adopt good brushing habits until after World War II, when veterans brought the concept of good oral health back to the United States!

THE PROS AND CONS OF BEING A DENTAL ASSISTANT

The dental assistant profession is healthy and growing, as you'll learn later in this chapter. If you choose to become a dental assistant, you'll likely have a wide range of possible settings and responsibilities. In addition to lots of opportunity, the dental assistant profession is stable and secure. The job demand is good, and the job is usually flexible. That means there are both full-time and part-time positions available. The working conditions are also considered quite good—dental offices are typically interesting, enjoyable, people-oriented environments.

Because it's practiced in many different settings, the day-to-day environment can vary greatly, which means you can find the kind of workplace that matches your needs and personality without leaving your profession. You can help to provide direct patient care in all sorts of dental specialties, including orthodontics, pediatric dentistry, periodontics, and oral surgery. Regardless of the setting, you'll work in a team-oriented environment, helping the dentists and working with hygienists and other assistants in the best interest of the patient.

Another advantage is that the pay is good in comparison to the amount of schooling required. However, dental assistants are usually paid the least compared to other dental-related professions. We talk about salaries more in the next section.

Despite its many advantages, there are a few "cons" to consider as well. One issue to keep in mind is the physicality of the job. You will be on your feet and working hands-on with patients all day. This can lead to chronic physical issues, such as back pain, neck and wrist pain, headaches, and numbness in the arms and wrists. Because dental assistants often need to work with X-ray machines, extra care must be taken to ensure that you remain safe and are not overexposed to harmful X-rays.

Another disadvantage is that dental assistants are typically the ones who have to clean up bodily fluids, such as blood and puss. If you're not ready to (safely) clean up patients' bodily fluids, this probably isn't the profession for you. As with all healthcare professions, there is always a risk of infection when working around patient populations. However, following basic safety procedures greatly diminishes this risk.

> "Don't get the idea that dental offices are free of bodily fluids—it's blood and puss. There are a lot of vessels in the mouth, which means there will be blood. If you can't handle that, you won't make it."—Adrienne Collins, dental hygienist

HOW HEALTHY IS THE DENTAL ASSISTANT JOB MARKET?

The Bureau of Labor Statistics is part of the US Department of Labor (see www.bls.gov). It tracks statistical information about thousands of careers in the United States. For anyone studying to become a dental assistant, the news is good! Employment is expected to grow 19 percent in the decade 2016 to

2026, which is faster than the average. Dental assistants, like many healthcare workers, are expected to be in great demand as the generation of baby boomers continues to age and struggle with health issues related to their teeth. In addition, recent studies have shown a link between oral health and general health, which is increasing patient demand for preventive dental services.

These statistics show just how promising this career is now and in the foreseeable future:[4]

- *Education:* Some states require a degree from an (Commission on Dental Accreditation) CODA-accredited program (from the ADA) and passing an exam. In other states, there are no formal educational requirements—dental assistants learn how to perform their jobs through on-the-job training.
- *2017 median pay:* $37,630
- *Job outlook 2016–2026:* 19 percent (faster than average)
- *Work environment:* Most work in a dental office setting (91 percent).

The jury is in: being a dental assistant is a stable and interesting career!

A DENTAL ASSISTANT IN A PERIODONTICS OFFICE

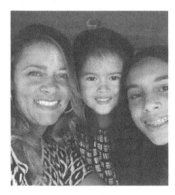

Lisa Alonso.
Courtesy of Lisa Alonso

Lisa Alonso (shown here with her two daughters) began working as an office assistant after high school for her own dentist. Her natural curiosity led her to the back of the office, where she began assisting the doctor. After four years, the dentist encouraged her to become licensed in the state of New York. She attended Hudson Valley Community College in Pennsylvania and became certified and licensed as a dental assistant in New York in 2005. In 2015, she moved to Florida and has worked in a periodontics office for three years.

Can you explain how you became interested in being a dental assistant and the specific educational process you went through?

The dentist who I worked for was my dentist. I was working for a pediatrician at the front desk and wanted to do something more. I wanted to be more hands-on. When I went to get a cleaning, my dentist told me they were hiring. They started me at the front desk. One day he was shorthanded, and that's where it all started. I asked a lot of questions and he saw that I wanted to learn. He asked if I wanted to move to the back. A year later, I became his main assistant. After four years, I took the test and became certified and licensed.

What is a typical day in your job?

The average day begins by preparing for the day. We check out the schedule and prepare records and papers. We do lots of surgeries and put patients under sedation, so we need to make sure we know of allergies, previous sedation records, and so on, for the doctor to be ready. We also prepare the operating room with instruments and equipment the doctor may need. With IV sedation, there is the doctor, the main chair assistant, a backup assistant (write medical prescriptions, check blood pressures, oxygen levels, and heart rates), and even a second backup assistant.

The surgeries are in the morning—usually three max. Patients can't eat 8 hours before if there is IV sedation, so patients want to be seen in the morning. Periodontists treat gums and bone issues—no crowns or fillings

Post-ops are in afternoon. We see patients after about a week of their surgery to check bone grafts, remove sutures, and make sure the patient is doing well.

We comfort patients and prepare them for dental procedures. We also communicate and educate patients about postsurgical procedures and instructions (eating, etc.). The hours are regular 8–5 days.

What's the best part of your job?

It's rewarding and fulfilling because it's challenging. It's fast-paced and no two days are the same. I get joy from caring for patients and helping them smile again or getting them out of pain, enhancing the quality of their life because now they can smile and feel better about themselves.

What's the worst part of your job?

For me, it's dealing with rude or mean patients who don't want to be there and take it out on you, when we are just trying to help them. That's hard sometimes.

Because of the way we work and position we sometimes stand in, it can be problematic for your back or neck, but you can sit or move around, which helps. I try sitting as much as I can while treating patients.

What's the most surprising thing about your job?

I guess how rewarding it is. Helping patients is very wonderful. Changing someone's face from worried and in pain to smiling and happy feels really good!

How has it changed since you started?

Technology has come a long way with digital X-rays, which are immediate instead of having to wait. Radiation is at a minimum, and there are new and better materials. New hand pieces, too. It has come a long way.

What's next—where do you see yourself going from here?

Truly, I like the field I am in. I like to help people. Whatever I do, I see myself still helping people as much as I can. I want to help them feel better about themselves.

What prepared you best for this job: the hands-on experience or the education and testing?

I definitely learned so much hands-on from my first dentist. I learn best by doing. The school was still very valuable. It teaches you about the field and prepares you for smooth transition to the actual workplace. They complement each other. You need both.

Is the job what you expected?

Yes, it is. One of my expectations was to have the opportunity to step into different roles and learn lots of different things, and I have been able to do that.

What would be your advice to a young person who is considering becoming a dental assistant?

You should want to help people. If you have diligence to learn technical and personal skills, that's good. You have to be a therapist to patients in a sense and talk to them about their problems and fears, etc., while they are there. People skills are important. If you love what you do, this becomes natural.

One nice thing is that you see instant results, which is great. The patients smile and are happy when they leave and are out of pain! If you like helping people so they can feel better about themselves, it's a very rewarding profession.

Try to get experience and visit dentists to make sure you can deal with blood and saliva. If you know you don't like blood, this is not the place for you.

DO YOU HAVE TO BE CERTIFIED OR LICENSED?

Although it is not legally required in every state, dental assistants are encouraged to become certified by passing an exam, as this shows potential employers and patients that they are capable of performing the duties required of them. Many places of employment (and certain states) might require this in order to be considered for a job. Most dental assistants become nationally certified by taking the Dental Assisting National Board's (DANB) Certified Dental Assistant (CDA) examination (see www .danb.org for more information). In order to sit for this exam, you must have completed a dental assisting program that is accredited by the Commission on Dental Accreditation—CODA (www.ada.org/en/coda). Chapter 3 covers in detail the educational requirements and explains how to find an accredited program near you.

Some states offer registration or licensure in addition to this national certification program. In order to determine the requirements in your state of residence, search the Internet for dental assistant license with your state's name. This is covered in more detail in chapter 3.

WOULD I BE A GOOD DENTAL ASSISTANT?

Ask yourself these questions:

- Am I comfortable touching people's mouths and teeth or could I learn to be comfortable with this idea?
- Am I comfortable cleaning up and working with bodily fluids, such as blood and puss?
- I am comfortable around people who are sick or have serious dental issues?

- Do I like meeting, talking with, and helping people? Do I consider myself a "people person"?
- Am I organized and reliable?
- Am I ready to spend most of my working day on my feet?
- Am I a lifelong learner and excited at the prospect of continuously learning?

"Patient interaction is my favorite part of being a dental assistant. I enjoy seeing people and knowing we made a difference. A patient initially comes in with really bad teeth and needs a debridement and now is doing amazing. They are coming back regularly and are appreciative. I like talking to the people. We know them when they come in."—Lisa Alonso, dental assistant

If the answer to any of these questions is an adamant no, you might want to consider a different path. Remember that learning what you don't like can be just as important and figuring out what you do like to do. If you think the dental profession is interesting, but want a little more responsibility, read on to learn about the dental hygienist.

What Is a Dental Hygienist?

Dental hygienists clean a patient's teeth and apply fluorides and sealants to teeth. They remove tartar, stains, and plaque as they brush, floss, and scrape. Dental hygienists also educate patients on the best ways to brush and floss teeth, as well as which products to use. They deal primarily with preventive healthcare for the teeth, whereas dentists more likely address problems that have occurred (cavities, etc.).

The dental hygienist career includes a wide range of responsibilities. The dentist and the dental hygienist work together to meet the oral health needs of their patients. States have different regulations, so the duties and tasks that dental hygienists perform depend on where you practice. However, responsibilities often include the following:[5]

- Patient screening procedures, such as assessment of oral health conditions, review of the health history, oral cancer screening, head and neck inspection, dental charting, and taking blood pressure and pulse rate
- Taking and developing dental X-rays
- Removing calculus and plaque (hard and soft deposits) from the teeth
- Applying preventive materials to the teeth (such as sealants and fluorides)
- Teaching patients proper oral hygiene strategies to maintain oral health (such as brushing and flossing)
- Educating patients about good nutrition and the impact on oral health
- Making impressions of patient teeth for casts

Dental hygienists can work in a variety of settings—including dentist offices, hospitals, schools, public health clinics, nursing facilities, and other healthcare facilities. Just like dental assistants, dental hygienists spend a lot of their time on their feet, working actively with patients.

Depending on your level of education and experience, you can also apply your skills and knowledge as a dental hygienist to other career activities, including teaching students in dental schools and dental hygiene education programs. Research, office management, and business administration are also career options. You may also find employment opportunities as a dental product sales representative working with companies that market dental-related materials and equipment.

> "My favorite thing about being a dental hygienist is when you win a frightened patient over. Initially they were scared and their oral health was poor, but now they come back regularly and are committed to taking care of their teeth. It feels good to know you helped make that happen."—Julia Guy, dental hygienist

Dental hygienists entering the profession usually need an associate's degree, which typically takes two years to complete. There are approximately 300 ADA-accredited dental hygiene education programs in community colleges, technical colleges, dental schools, and universities in the United States.[6] Visit the ADA website's listing of accredited programs to find a good one close to you (see www.ada.org/en/coda/find-a-program).

Chapters 2 and 3 cover the educational and professional certification requirements in more detail.

THE PROS AND CONS OF BEING A DENTAL HYGIENIST

Being a dental hygienist provides many rewards. Many dental hygienists report that one of the most fulfilling and enjoyable parts of the job is working with people every day. They enjoy talking to and getting to know their patients, helping to calm them and allay their fears, and even becoming friends with some and being inspired by others. Personal fulfillment also comes from providing an important healthcare service while establishing trusting relationships with patients.

Dental hygienists also enjoy the flexibility that their profession offers. There are full-time and part-time employment options as well as evening and weekend hours, which can enable you to balance your career and lifestyle demands. Some offices offer eight-hour days, whereas others allow for four ten-hour days and other options. Hygienists also have opportunities to work in many different situations, including private dental practices, educational and community institutions, research teams, and dental corporations. In addition to flexible schedules, there is a lot of variety in this profession. Patients don't have a one-size-fits-all solution to their oral issues, and dental hygienists play an important role in addressing all kinds of interpersonal and clinical hurdles to health. This job is never boring!

There is security in this profession as well, as the services they provide are needed and valued by a large part of the population. Current demand is high and there will be excellent opportunities into the future as well.

Despite its many advantages, there are a few "cons" to consider as well. One issue to keep in mind is the physicality of the job. You will be on your feet and working hands-on with your patients all day. This can lead to chronic physical issues, such as back, neck, and wrist pain, that you need to be ready to manage and treat yourself. Many dental hygienists make it a point to get massages regularly.

Another challenge is working with patients who don't comply with treatment or who aren't properly educated about oral health and don't seem willing to make a change. Seeing children who suffer due to their parents' lack of knowledge can be especially difficult. However, as with all challenges, this can be extremely rewarding as well, when you and your team do make a difference in someone's life.

Finally, as with all healthcare professions, there is always a risk of infection when working around patient populations, especially if you work in a hospital, nursing home, or healthcare facility.

DID GEORGE WASHINGTON REALLY HAVE WOODEN TEETH?

Despite the urban legend, our first president did not actually have wooden teeth. He did have long-standing dental problems, though, and by the time he became the first US president at age 57, it was reported that he had only one real tooth left in his mouth. He had several pairs of dentures throughout his life, although none of them were wooden. The dentures he wore at his inauguration were made by Dr. John Greenwood, known has the "Father of Modern Dentistry," and were carved from hippopotamus ivory, lead, and human and animal teeth—including horse and donkey teeth. One pair was later donated to the Smithsonian.[7]

HOW HEALTHY IS THE DENTAL HYGIENIST JOB MARKET?

The Bureau of Labor Statistics is part of the US Department of Labor (see www.bls.gov). It tracks statistical information about thousands of careers in the United States. For anyone studying to become a dental hygienist, the news is good! Employment is expected to grow 20 percent in the decade 2016 to 2026, which is much faster than the average. Dental hygienists, like many healthcare workers, are expected to be in great demand as the generation of baby boomers continues to age and struggle with health issues related to their teeth. In addition, recent studies have shown a link between oral health and general health, which is increasing patient demand for preventive dental services.

These statistics show just how promising this career is now and in the foreseeable future:[8]

- *Education:* Associate's degree. All states require dental hygienists to be licensed, although the requirements vary by state.
- *2017 median pay:* $74,074
- *Job outlook 2016–2026:* 20 percent (much faster than average)
- *Work environment:* Most (95 percent) work in private dental offices.

WOULD I BE A GOOD DENTAL HYGIENIST?

Ask yourself these questions:

- Am I comfortable touching people's mouths and teeth or could I learn to be comfortable with this idea?
- Am I comfortable cleaning up and working with bodily fluids, such as blood and puss?
- I am comfortable around people who are sick or have serious dental issues?
- Do I like meeting, talking with, and helping people? Do I consider myself a "people person"?
- Am I organized and reliable?
- Am I ready to spend most of my working day on my feet?
- Am I a lifelong learner and excited at the prospect of continuously learning?

If the answer to any of these questions is an adamant no, you might want to consider a different path. Remember that learning what you don't like can be just as important and figuring out what you do like to do. If you think the dental profession is interesting, but you aren't crazy about the idea of interacting with patients directly, read on to learn about being a dental technician.

What Is a Dental Laboratory Technician?

A dental technician (also called a dental laboratory technician) works behind the scenes, usually in a laboratory setting, creating custom-made dental appliances such as dentures, dental bridges, crowns, braces, and implants from instructions they receive from the dentist. This is considered a science and an art, because each patient's needs are different and your creations must be tailored for their mouth. Dental technicians typically do not work directly with patients.

Dental technicians may create any of the following from impressions of the teeth and oral soft tissues:

- Crowns, which are caps designed to restore the size and shape of an injured tooth
- Veneers, which enhance the look and function of the teeth

- Removable partial dentures or fixed bridges for patients who are missing a few teeth
- Orthodontic appliances to help straighten and protect teeth
- Full dentures for patients who are missing all of their teeth

Dental technicians are at the forefront of promising new technologies and materials. They work with many different materials, including waxes, plastics, precious and nonprecious alloys, stainless steel, and porcelains and composites. Dental technicians have marketable skills, because they can use sophisticated instruments and equipment.

The work environment varies, depending on whether you work for a commercial lab or for a private dentist office. The majority of dental technicians in the United States work in commercial dental laboratories. The average laboratory employs about five to ten technicians. Some dental technicians provide a whole range of dental prosthetic services, whereas others specialize in one particular type (such as removable partial dentures, crown and bridge, veneers, and so on).[9]

If you want to work more closely one-on-one with a dentist, there are opportunities to work in private dental offices as well. A smaller percentage of dental technicians work in dental schools, hospitals, and companies that manufacture dental prosthetic materials.

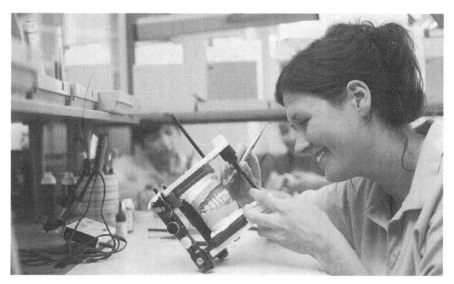

Dental technicians work in a laboratory setting creating custom-made dental appliances.

THE PROS AND CONS OF THE DENTAL TECHNICIAN FIELD

Consider the following characteristics of the career. What might be a disadvantage to some is an advantage to another, so it's a good idea to know what you want and need out of a career as you learn and read about each profession:

- *Flexibility:* There are several different settings and lots of different opportunities for advancement. You can work in a commercial laboratory, where the pay is best, and work your way up to a supervisory role, or even own your own laboratory over time.
- *Independence:* You will typically be able to do most of your work without close supervision. Because you "own" each project from start to finish, you'll likely experience the satisfaction that comes from creating something from scratch, especially when it will help someone.
- *Creativity:* Creating dentures and appliances for patients requires an artistic skill and creativity, which can be very fulfilling but also demanding. Fine-motor skills and excellent hand-eye coordination are a must.
- *Job security:* With the baby-boomer population growing older, there will be a continued and increased demand for dental prostheses. Recent improvements in technology and materials that resulted in reduced costs have also increased demand for restorative and cosmetic dentistry. The ADA expects that employment opportunities in the dental technician field will be excellent well into the next century.
- *Physically demanding:* As with many jobs in dentistry and healthcare in general, this is a job that requires a lot of physical stamina to do well. Even though you do have more opportunity to sit than a dental hygienist might, dental technicians still deal with repetitive stress injuries sometimes. You must have very good arm-hand steadiness and excellent near vision.
- *Pays well:* The pay is good, especially compared to the small amount of formal education required to do it. In fact, most dental laboratory technicians learn their craft through on-the-job training. They typically begin as helpers in the laboratory and learn more advanced skills as they gain experience.

DENTAL LABORATORY TECHNICIAN SPECIALTY AREAS

Depending on your personal interests, you can focus your creative efforts on one of any of the following:

- Orthodontics (braces, retainers, and other corrective devices)
- Implants, which are placed into bone
- Porcelain and ceramic veneers, placed over an injured or unsightly tooth
- Dentures, full and partial
- Crowns (caps over damaged teeth)
- Bridges (dental devices that replace missing teeth by joining an artificial tooth to nearby teeth or dental implants)

HOW HEALTHY IS THE DENTAL TECHNICIAN JOB MARKET?

The Bureau of Labor Statistics (see www.bls.gov) tracks statistical information about thousands of careers in the United States. According to their statistics, the US job market for a dental laboratory technician is expected to grow 13 percent in the decade from 2016 to 2026, which is faster than average. As mentioned previously, job demand is healthy due to an increasing elderly population requiring more services and the increasing demand for affordable restorative and cosmetic dentistry.

These statistics show just how promising this career is now and in the foreseeable future:[10]

- *Education:* On-the-job training
- *2016 median pay:* $35,250
- *Job outlook 2016–2026:* 13 percent (faster than average)
- *Work environment:* Most work in laboratory settings, full time. Many also work for private dentist offices.

WOULD I BE A GOOD DENTAL TECHNICIAN?

Ask yourself these questions:

- Am I comfortable learning on the job, without a lot of formal schooling?

- Do I have very good fine-motor skills, good hand-eye coordination, and arm-hand steadiness?
- Do I have good near vision?
- Am I a detail-oriented person?
- Am I a creative person who enjoys crafting with my hands?
- Am I an independently motivated person? Can I make deadlines without being closely supervised?
- Am I ready to spend most of my working day in a physical job?
- Am I a lifelong learner and excited at the prospect of continuously learning?

If the answer to any of these questions is an adamant no, you might want to consider a different path. Fortunately, dental technicians and dental hygienists (and assistants) are complementary professions, so if you're not cut out for one, it's likely you'll be well suited for the other.

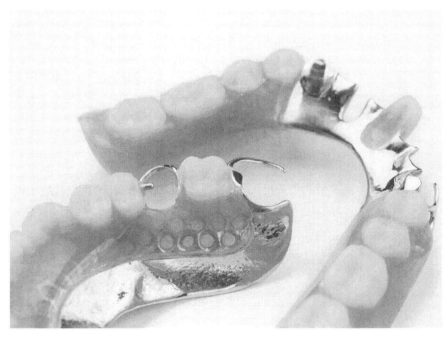

Because of the availability of cheaper and better materials, there has been an increased demand for restorative and cosmetic dentistry.

CHARACTERISTICS OF SUCCESS IN THE DENTAL HEALTH FIELDS

Regardless of the profession you choose in dental health, there are commonalities that all people who enjoy success in these areas share. Consider how well the following phrases describe who you are:

- Enjoy helping people
- Enjoy cooperative and collaborative work
- Feel comfortable working in people's mouths
- Feel comfortable motivating others
- Empathetic toward pain and suffering
- Get energy from being around others

The caveat here is that you can be a good dental laboratory technician and not be expected to work with patients and the public in general. However, you will still need to communicate effectively with dentists and other professionals and co-workers. Remember that if you pursue a career that fundamentally conflicts with the person you are, you won't be good at it and you won't be happy. Don't make that mistake. Need help in determining your key personality factors? Take a career counseling questionnaire to find out more. You can find many online or ask you school guidance counselor for reputable sources.

Summary

In this chapter, you learned a lot about the different careers in the dental health umbrella—dental assistants, dental hygienists, and dental technicians. You've learned about what people in these professions do in their day-to-day work, the environments where you can find these people working, some pros and cons about each career path, the average salaries of these jobs, and the outlook in the future for all these careers. You hopefully even contemplated some questions about whether your personal likes and preferences meld well with these jobs. At this time, you should have a good idea what each job looks like. Are you starting to get excited about one field over another? If not, that's okay, as there's still time.

An important takeaway from this chapter is that no matter which of these professions you might pursue, keep in mind that maintaining current certifications and meeting the continuing education requirements is very important in all health-related careers. Advances in understanding in the fields of medicine, nutrition, and more are continuous, and it's vitally important that you keep apprised of what's happening if your field. You need to have a lifelong love of learning to succeed in any dental health career.

In chapter 2, we dive into forming a plan for your future. We cover everything there is to know about educational requirements, certifications, internship and clinical requirements, and more, about each of these careers. You'll learn about finding summer jobs and making the most of volunteer work as well. The goal is for you to set yourself apart—and above—the rest.

2

Forming a Career Plan

Now that you have some idea which career you want to find out more about, or maybe you even know which one you will start pursuing, it's time to formulate a career plan. For you organized folks out there, this can be a helpful and energizing process. If you're not a naturally organized person, or perhaps the idea of looking ahead and building a plan to adulthood scares you, you are not alone. That's what this chapter is for.

After we talk about ways to develop a career plan (there is more than one way to do this!), the chapter dives into the various educational requirements of these professions. Finally, we will look at how you can gain experience through internships, volunteering, clinic work, shadowing, and more. Yes, experience will look good on your resume and in some cases it's even required. But even more important, getting out there and experiencing a job in various settings is the best way to determine if it's really something that you will enjoy or not. When you find a career that you truly enjoy, it will rarely feel like work at all.

If you still aren't sure which of these professions, if any, is right for you, try a self-assessment questionnaire or a career aptitude test. There are many good ones on the web. As an example, the career-resource website Monster.com includes its favorite free self-assessment tools at www.monster.com/career-advice/article/best-free-career-assessment-tools. The Princeton Review also has a very good aptitude test geared toward high schoolers at www.princetonreview.com/quiz/career-quiz.

Your ultimate goal should be to match your personal interests/goals with your preparation plan for college/careers. Practice articulating your plans and goals to others. Once you feel comfortable doing this, that means you have a good grasp of your goals and the plan to reach them.

Planning the Plan

You are on a fact-finding mission of sorts. A career fact-finding plan, no matter what the field, should include these main steps:

- Take some time to consider and jot down your interests and personality traits. Are you a people person or do you get energy from being alone? Are you creative or analytical? Are you outgoing or shy? Are you organized or creative, or a little of both? Take a career-counseling questionnaire (found online or in your guidance counselor's office) to find out more. Consider whether your personal likes and preferences meld well with the jobs you are considering.
- Find out as much as you can about the day-to-day of the job. In what kinds of environments is it performed? Who will you work with? How demanding is the job? What are the challenges? Chapter 1 of this book is designed to help you in this regard.
- Find out about educational requirements and schooling expectations. Will you be able to meet any rigorous requirements? This chapter will help you understand the educational paths and licensing requirements of these professions.
- Seek out opportunities to volunteer or shadow professionals doing the job. Use your critical thinking skills to ask questions and consider whether this is the right environment for you. This chapter also discusses ways to find internships, summer jobs, and other job-related experiences.
- Look into student aid, grants, scholarships, and other ways you can get help to pay for schooling. It's not just about student aid and scholarships, either. Some larger organizations will pay employees to go back to school to get further degrees.
- Build a timetable for taking requirements exams such as the SAT and ACT, applying to schools, visiting schools, and making your decision. You should write down all important deadlines and have them at the ready when you need them.
- Continue to look for employment that matters during your college years—internships and work experiences that help you build hands-on experience and knowledge about your actual career.

- Find a mentor who is currently practicing in your field of interest. This person can be a great source of information, education, and connections. Don't expect a job (at least not at first); just build a relationship with someone who wants to pass along their wisdom and experience. Coffee meetings or even e-mails are a great way to start.

> "I took a vocational class and then shadowed my hygienist. It helped me to know if I could actually handle the job. I would recommend that students get all the info they can and talk to other hygienists. Meet the doctors and see what they are like too."—Lindsey Jones, dental hygienist

Where to Go for Help

If you aren't sure where to start, your local library, school library, and guidance counselor office are great places to begin. Search your local or school library

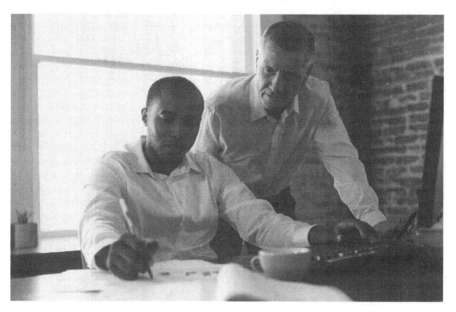

A mentor can help you figure out which way to go with your career aspirations.

for resources about finding a career path and finding the right schooling that fits your needs and budget. Make an appointment with a counselor or e-mail them and ask about taking career interest questionnaires. With a little prodding, you'll be directed to lots of good information online and elsewhere. You can start your research with these four sites:

- The Bureau of Labor Statistics' Career Outlook site at https://www.bls .gov/careeroutlook/home.htm. The United States Department of Labor's Bureau of Labor Statistics site doesn't just track job statistics, as you learned in chapter 1. There is an entire portion of this site dedicated to young adults looking to uncover their interests and match those interests with jobs currently in the market. There is a section called "Career Planning for High Schoolers" that you should check out. Information is updated based on career trends and jobs in demand, so you'll get practice information as well.
- The Mapping Your Future site at www.mappingyourfuture.org helps you determine a career path and then helps you map out a plan to reach those goals. It includes tips on preparing for college, paying for college, job hunting, résumé writing, and more.
- The Education Planner site at www.educationplanner.org has separate sections for students, parents, and counselors. It breaks down the task of planning your career goals into simple, easy-to-understand steps. You can find personality assessments, get tips for preparing for school, learn from some Q&As from counselors, download and use a planner worksheet, read about how to finance your education, and more.
- TeenLife at www.teenlife.com calls itself "the leading source for college preparation" and it includes lots of information about summer programs, gap year programs, community service, and more. They believe that spending time out "in the world" outside of the classroom can help students do better in school, find a better fit in terms of career, and even interview better with colleges. This site contains lots of links to volunteer and summer programs.

Use these sites as jumping off points and don't be afraid to reach out to a real person, such as a guidance counselor, if you're feeling overwhelmed.

BEING A DENTAL HYGIENIST IN A GENERAL PRACTICE SETTING

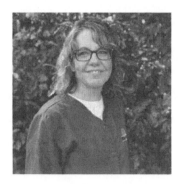

Catherine Kimmey. *Courtesy of Catherine Kimmey*

Catherine Kimmey received her associate of science degree in 2001 from the University of New England, Portland, Maine. She has worked in a general practice dentistry setting her entire career, first in Maine and then in Maryland. She became interested in dental hygiene as a career after reading a career book in high school.

What is a typical day in your job?

I work in a general practice setting, so I see many different types of patients, ages three to late nineties. I provide prophylaxis (fancy word for cleaning), take X-rays, do periodontal probings to determine the health of someone's mouth, and do scaling and root planings for patients with more advanced decay. These kinds of therapies run about 50 minutes. I also treat infections, give fluoride, apply sealants, and provide other maintenance to stop progression of disease and infection. Adult (14 and up) visits are usually 50 minutes, children (5 and up) are 40 minutes, and kids under 5 are 30 minutes. The hours are usually flexible and you can do morning shifts or evening shifts. You can even pick days you work and you can work part-time.

The flexibility is nice. Our office has morning and afternoon shifts, as well as shifts of different lengths. So you can usually find something that works well with your life and other obligations. I prefer working 10-hour days when I can. So I usually work three 10-hour days and one eight-hour day as a full-time dental hygienist. And it's not a job behind the desk, which appealed to me.

During their visits, I also talk to patients about cleaning, how to take care of your mouth, how disease in your mouth affects your entire body, how to keep your teeth and gums healthy, and other preventative measures. A large part of my job is education.

Hygienists are considered providers, so we work closely with doctors. It's important that we can work well with others. Hygienists should be friendly and likable (compassionate and understanding) and want to help patients who are nervous and don't like going to the dentist.

What's the best part of your job?

The people. I love being around patients. I get to meet a lot of interesting people from all different backgrounds that have had amazing lives. My favorite age range, I guess, is adults because they can converse well during the visit. I also really like the people I work with.

Bringing someone with bad oral health to a place of good oral health is also very satisfying. In addition, the pay scale is good, and there is lots of flexibility.

What's the worst part of your job?

The toll it takes on your body. There is a lot of repetitive motion. You are in positions that aren't really great for your muscles. You'll see a lot of hygienists and dentist with hunched shoulders, due to basically how we work. Being in the specific positions to make patients comfortable can be hard on your shoulders, neck, back, and wrists. It puts you at a pretty high risk for injuries if you don't take care of yourself. Exercise and stretching is important, as is making sure you have the proper equipment. Massages—at least on your neck and shoulders— once a month are a good idea. Loosen your muscles. Having a good, strong core helps, too.

What's the most surprising thing about your job?

When in school, you have a quite a bit of time for your patients. You have one to two patients a day. But then you get to work, and you have 50 minutes for patients. But it does all come together. It's really a team-oriented environment—that was surprising to me. You help each other out and work together so much more than I realized. This includes the dentist, the front desk, other hygienists, and dental assistants. You work with them all together.

What's next? Where do you see yourself going from here?

I am happy where I am. But if you want growth in a career setting, you could get your masters and teach. Or, if you're in a bigger practice with multiple locations, you can become manager, etc. I really love my job and want to continue doing it. I would like to work fewer hours eventually, as I get closer to retirement.

Did your education prepare you for the job?

Absolutely—I had a great group of professors who wanted to make sure we were prepared. Hands-on and approachable professors. They prepared us for our exams, too.

Mine was a three-year program, although some programs exist that are shorter and require summer classes. We even had an "office manager" who scheduled our patients. The first couple of semesters were all classroom, to get the prerequisites out of the way. The second and third years are spent in the clinic, with a few classes as well. Lots of labs and clinic time. There are X-ray classes, anesthesia courses, etc. You practice on each other as well before patients. I saw patients for about three semesters. These are typically people without insurance—lots of kids and retirees and students. Your requirements are to see so many patients that are adults, so many as kids, so many bitewings, so many cleanings, so many sealants, etc.

Is the job what you expected?

For the most part, yes. One surprise is that I didn't realize how many people had dental anxiety, because I wasn't scared of the dentist myself. I didn't see that part in dental school. Nitrous gas helps. Oral sedation also helps. Also, the teamwork aspect surprised me, but I really enjoy that.

Any advice for young people thinking about going into this field?

Study hard. This is a really great job where you get to meet so many different people. Some of those will inspire your life; some of those people will become your friends. If you are a people person, it's a great environment to work in.

If you aren't sure if you would like working with people's teeth and bodily fluids, job shadow and see if you can deal with it and like it. A lot of people who want to become dental hygienists come and work behind us and see what our job entails. That's common and many schools even make you do that before you can apply. You can also enter the field more easily as a dental assistant and work for a while to see if you want to become a hygienist.

Making High School Count

Regardless of the career you choose, if you are interested in dental health, there are some basic yet important things you can do while in high school to position yourself in the most advantageous way. Remember—it's not just about having the best application, it's also about figuring out what professions you actually would enjoy doing and which ones don't suit you.

- Load up on the sciences, especially biology and anatomy. A head start in anatomy, biology, and/or physiology will be a big help.
- Sign up for psychology. You treat the whole person, not just a body.
- Be comfortable using all kinds of computer software.
- Learn first aid and CPR. You'll need these important skills regardless of your profession.
- Hone your communication skills in English, speech, and debate. You'll need them to speak with everyone from dentists to patients in pain.
- Volunteer in as many settings as you can. Read on to learn more about this important aspect of career planning.

Educational Requirements

The nice thing is that no matter what degree of postsecondary education you can/want to pursue, there is a way for you to choose a profession in dental health if that is your passion. The following sections cover each profession discussed so far in more detail.

EDUCATIONAL REQUIREMENTS FOR A DENTAL ASSISTANT

There are two main paths you can follow to become a dental assistant, depending on the state in which you live—by graduating from an accredited program and receiving certification or by learning on-the-job. There are currently 15 states that require some type of training for dental assistants, whereas a few states—including Minnesota, California, and Michigan—have even more specific educational standards and examinations for their registered dental assistants.[1]

Many states still have no training, credentialing, or continued education standards for dental assistants. In states not yet requiring such certification, dental assistants often learn how to perform their jobs through on-the-job training. However, you may still be required to be certified if you want to perform special functions, such as take X-rays, depending on the state.

> **Tip:** Although it is not legally required in every state, becoming certified as a dental assistant shows potential employers and patients that you are capable of performing the duties required. Many places of employment (and certain states) might require certification in order to be considered for a job.

The Commission on Dental Accreditation (CODA), part of the American Dental Association (ADA), accredited nearly three hundred dental assisting training programs in 2017. An accredited program is one that has been vetted by the ADA/CODA through peer reviews and on-site reviews and has been proven to meet the minimum accreditation quality standards. Most programs are offered through community colleges, although you can also find accredited programs through vocational or technical schools.

> "I definitely learned so much hands-on from my first dentist. I learn best by doing. But the schooling was still very valuable. It teaches you about the field and prepares you for smooth transition to the actual workplace. They complement each other. You need both."—Lisa Alonso, dental assistant

These programs usually take about one year to complete, after which you receive a certificate or diploma. There are also programs that last two years and lead to an associate's degree, but they are less common. An associate's degree could make you more marketable in the long run, especially if you think you may work in different states. See www.ada.org/en/coda for a fully searchable listing of accredited schools in your area.

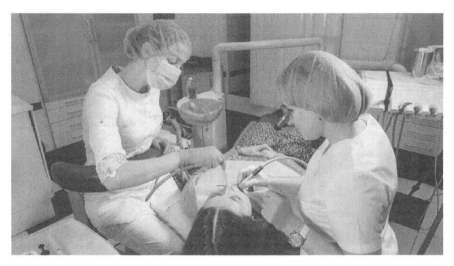

During your dental assistant training, you will gain supervised practical experience.

Dental assistant programs are a mix of classroom and laboratory work. You will learn about teeth and gums, as well as other areas that dentists work on and the instruments that dentists use. These programs also include supervised practical experience.

Entry-Level Requirements for Dental Assistants

If your state allows it, you can enter the workforce as a dental assistant in training and learn on the job while earning a salary. Many states use specific titles for these kinds of dental assistants in training. For example, in California, they are called "unlicensed dental assistants," and in Iowa they are called "dental assistant trainees."[2] In these cases, you must satisfactorily complete a probationary time period before you can apply for your license/registration or begin performing additional functions.

If your state has no requirements, dental assistants are allowed to perform basic supportive dental procedures (in the presence of and supporting the dentist or hygienist) without completing specific training requirements. However, the more experience and training you have in areas like infection control, radiology, and intraoral procedures, the more marketable you will be and the easier it will be to find a position.

Note: Radiology requirements (to take dental X-rays) are a good example of something that varies greatly from state to state. Some states, such as New York State and Alaska, have no radiography requirements for dental assistants, which typically means that dental assistants cannot operate dental X-ray equipment unless directly supervised by a registered dentist.

Many states—such as Florida, Indiana, and California—have specific requirements for dental assistants who operate dental X-ray equipment and perform dental radiographic procedures. Dental assistants sometimes must pass a safety exam or radiology exam, or must successfully complete a dental radiography training program. As you can see, it's important to understand the requirements of the state in which you plan to live and work before you map out your educational plans. However, graduating from a CODA-accredited program benefits you no matter where you live in the United States.

As an example of what you can expect, here are some examples of basic requirements for *beginning* (not registered) dental assistants in various states:

- Washington: A seven-hour AIDS education course
- Vermont: Emergency procedures training within 180 days of being hired
- South Dakota: High school diploma and minimum age 18
- Mississippi: CPR certification within 180 days of employment
- Minnesota: CPR certification
- California: The completion of a state course after four months of training

In almost all these cases above, you will move to a licensed or registered dental assistant position after a certain number of hours worked and with successful completion of the required certifications.

Note: You can get more information about dental assistant state requirements from these websites:

The DALE Foundation maintains information on state requirements compiled by the Dental Assisting National Board (DANB) and state dental boards. See www.dalefoundation.org/Resources-And-State-Requirements/State-Dental-Assistant-Requirements.

The DANB also maintains current state information on its website and provides links to the appropriate state Boards of Dental Examiners. See www.danb.org/Meet-State-Requirements.aspx.

EDUCATIONAL REQUIREMENTS FOR DENTAL HYGIENISTS

In order to be able to practice as a dental hygienist, you need to earn an associate's degree from an accredited program in dental hygiene, which usually takes about three years to complete. In addition, all states also require dental hygienists to be licensed, but the requirements for licensing vary by state. Licensing is discussed more shortly.

Although the associate's degree is the most common path, there are also bachelor's and even master's degree programs in dental hygiene. A bachelor's or master's degree is often required for research, teaching, or clinical practice in public or school health programs.

Dental hygiene programs are commonly found in community colleges, technical schools, and universities. In 2017, CODA (part of the ADA) accredited more than three hundred dental hygiene programs. See www.ada.org/en/coda for a fully searchable listing of accredited schools in your area.

Accredited programs are a mix of classroom, laboratory, and clinical instruction. Areas of study include physiology, nutrition, radiography, pathology, medical ethics, anatomy, patient management, and periodontics (the study of gum disease).

Getting Your Dental Hygienist License

In nearly every state, you need to complete the following steps before you can apply for a dental hygienist license:

- You must graduate from an accredited dental hygiene program, as explained in the previous section.
- You must pass the written National Board Dental Hygiene Examination (NDBHE), which is discussed shortly.
- You must pass a regional or state clinical board examination, depending on your state's requirements, which is also discussed shortly.

It's important to remember that licensing requirements are different from state to state, so your best bet is to contact the licensing authority in your state for the specifics. To maintain licensure, you also will have to complete continuing education requirements.

> **Note:** For the specific requirements in your state, check out www.dentalcareersedu.org/how-to-become-a-dental-hygienist. It includes a clickable map that provides detailed information about each state's exams and requirements to practice as a dental hygienist.

National Board Examination

The Joint Commission on National Dental Examinations (JCNDE; see www.ada.org/en/jcnde) is the agency responsible for creating and administering the written tests for dentists and dental hygienists. The current written exam for dental hygienists is called the National Board Dental Hygiene Examination (NBDHE). A passing score is usually 75 percent or above.

> **Note:** The JCNDE is currently developing an updated test, called the Integrated National Board Dental Examination (INBDE), which will be available no sooner than 2020.

The purpose of the NBDHE/INBDE is to help state boards verify the qualifications of dental hygienists who want a license to practice dental hygiene in their states. This written exam assesses your ability to understand basic biomedical and dental sciences information and apply that information in context.

EXAMPLE NBDHE EXAM QUESTIONS

To give you a feel for the type and format of the NBDHE/INBDE test, the following are old example questions. In addition to multiple choice, there are also case histories that you read and then answer multiple questions about. You might even be given X-rays that you have to answer questions about.

The virus responsible for which of the following diseases is the MOST resistant to chemical and physical agents?

    A. AIDS   D. Influenza
    B. Herpes   E. Hepatitis
    C. Measles

Root hypersensitivity diminishes as the tooth forms which of the following?

    A. Mantle dentin   C. Cellular cementum
    B. Secondary dentin   D. Acellular cementum

The answers are hepatitis and cellular cementum, in case you're curious.

Regional Board Examinations (CDCA, SRTA, CRDTS, or WREB)

In most cases, you will also be required to pass a regional clinical exam in order to receive a license to practice dental hygiene in the state in which you live. These are clinical exams, which means you are working on actual patients and providing skill-specific treatment, while being assessed by third parties. A passing grade is usually 75 percent or above.

The purpose of these clinical regional boards is to make the licensure process more clear for candidates and eliminate the need for multiple state board clinical examinations. Fees for these exams range from $750 to $1,000.

Many states are associated with more than one regional board, which are listed here:

- CDCA (Commission on Dental Competency Assessments, previously the North East Regional Board, or NERB) includes twenty-four states in its jurisdiction, from Maine and Florida to Hawaii.
- CRDTS (Central Regional Dental Testing Service) includes the state boards of Alabama, Arkansas, California, Georgia, Hawaii, Illinois, Iowa, Kansas, Minnesota, Missouri, Nebraska, New Mexico, North Dakota, Oklahoma, South Carolina, South Dakota, Texas, Washington, West Virginia, Wisconsin, and Wyoming in its jurisdiction.
- CITA (Council of Interstate Testing Agencies) includes the state boards of Alabama, Louisiana, North Carolina, and West Virginia.
- SRTA (Southern Regional Testing Agency) includes the state boards of Alabama, Arkansas, South Carolina, Tennessee, Virginia, and West Virginia.
- WREB (Western Region Examining Board) includes the states of California, Oregon, Utah, Arizona, Idaho, Minnesota, Oklahoma, Texas, and Washington.

For a visual overview of the regional boards and which states are covered, check out the following table from the American Dental Hygienists Association (www.adha.org/licensure).

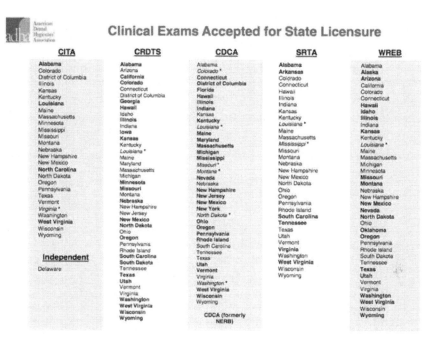

List of regional boards' clinical exams; states in bold are registered members.
Source: American Dental Hygenists Association, "Licensure," www.adha.org/licensure

EDUCATIONAL REQUIREMENTS FOR DENTAL LAB TECHNICIANS

Most dental laboratory technicians learn their trade from on-the-job training. They usually begin as assistants in the laboratory and learn more advanced skills as they get experience. For example, technicians in training might begin by pouring plaster into an impression, and then eventually move to more complicated jobs, such as making porcelain crowns or bridges. Because all laboratories are different, the length of training varies.[3] A few businesses in some states also sponsor registered apprenticeship training for dental laboratory technicians.

A high school diploma, lots of persistence, and maybe a personal connection, is usually enough to get an entry-level position as a dental laboratory technician. You can make the most of your high school years by taking courses in science, mathematics, computer programming, and art.

You can also pursue dental technician training through a two-year program at a community college, vocational school, technical college, university, or dental school. In most cases, you simply need a high school diploma or the equivalent to apply to an accredited dental laboratory technology program.

You'll receive a short-term certificate or a two-year associate's degree from these programs. These training programs usually include courses in dental anatomy, dental ceramics, and dentures; they sometimes also offer programs in management and business, which can help you in the long run if you're thinking about opening your own dental appliances manufacturing business. There also are a few programs out there that offer a four-year program in dental technology.

> **Note:** Dental appliance laboratories are creating more and more of their dental devices using advanced computer programs, so you may also want to take courses and gain experience in computer skills and programming.

To date, the ADA has accredited more than 20 programs in dental laboratory technology from community colleges and other postsecondary schools (see www.ada.org for the most updated current list).

Certification

Once you graduate from a program or are working as a dental lab technician, you can become a certified dental technician (CDT) by passing an examination that evaluates your technical skills and knowledge. The examination, which has written and clinical/practical parts, is administered by the National Board for Certification in Dental Laboratory Technology (NBC). Certified dental technicians specialize in one or more of these six areas: implants, complete dentures, removable partial dentures, crown and bridge, ceramics, or orthodontics.

See the NBC website at nbccert.org/homepage.cfm for current certification requirements.

> **Note:** Before you go through the process of being certified as a CDT, ask around your region and state to see if this extra effort and cost will benefit you in terms of career advancement and pay. Answers may vary depending on your state and the type of lab where you work.

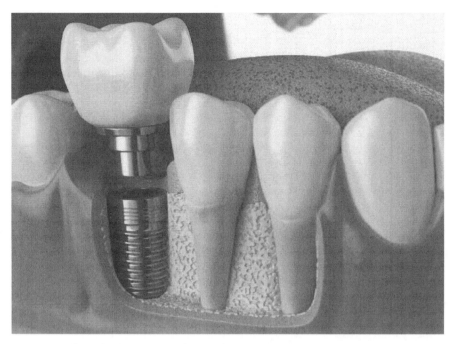

Dental implants are one of the appliances you may be required to create or modify for a patient's mouth.

Experience-Related Requirements

This section covers the required fieldwork of each profession, which is the fieldwork and/or internship work you'll do during the course of earning your degree or certifications. It also discusses other ways you can get experience in the dental field before and during the time you're pursuing your education. This can and should start in middle school or high school, especially during the summers. Experience is important for many reasons, not the least:

- Shadowing others in the profession can help reveal what the job is really like and whether it's something that you think you want to do, day in and day out. This is a relatively risk-free way to explore different career paths. Ask any "seasoned" adult and they will tell you that figuring out what you *don't* want to do is sometimes more important than figuring out what you *do* want to do.

- Internships and volunteer work are a relatively quick way to gain work experience and develop job skills.
- Volunteering can help you learn the intricacies of the profession, such as what types of environments are best, what kind of care fits you better, and which areas are in more demand.
- Gaining experience during your high school years sets you apart from the many others who are applying to programs.
- Volunteering in the field means that you'll be meeting many others doing the job that you might someday want to do (think: career networking). You have the potential to develop mentor relationships, cultivate future job prospects, and get to know people who can recommend you for later positions. Studies show that about 85 percent of jobs are found through personal contacts.[4]

Experience can come in the form of volunteering at the local clinic or in your community, taking on an internship in the summer, finding a summer job that complements your interests, or even attending camps that foster your career aspirations (see www.teenlife.com to start). Consider these tidbits of advice to maximize your volunteer experience.[5] They will help you stand out in competitive fields:

- Get diverse experiences. For example, try to shadow in at least two different dentists offices of differing sizes and specialties.
- Try to gain forty hours of volunteer experience in each setting. This is typically considered enough to show that you understand what a full workweek looks like in that setting. This can be as few as four to five hours per week over ten weeks or so.
- If your profession has such a job, find an aide/tech position. Working as a paid aide is by far the best experience you can get. This will prepare you nicely for your clinical experiences and tests as well.
- Don't be afraid to ask questions. Just be considerate of the professionals' time and wait until they are not busy to pursue your questions. Asking good questions shows that you have a real curiosity for the profession.
- Maintain and cultivate professional relationships. Write thank you notes, send updates about your application progress and tell them where you decide to go to school, and check in occasionally. If you want to find a good mentor, you need to be a gracious and willing mentee.

GETTING EXPERIENCE IN THE DENTAL HYGIENIST AND DENTAL ASSISTANT FIELDS

If you're currently in high school and you're seriously thinking about becoming a dental assistant or hygienist, start by reaching out to your own dentist or orthodontist, or to a family friend who runs or works in a dental office. Start by asking good questions and showing your curiosity. Ask to shadow the assistants and hygienists, remembering the guidelines about courtesy above. Don't expect to be paid for any of this effort at first. The benefit of volunteering is that it's much easier to get your foot in the door, but the drawback is that you typically will not be paid. However, with time and hard work, your volunteer position may turn into something else.

Look at these kinds of experiences as ways to learn about the profession. It may even help you to get into the program of your choice, and it will definitely help you write your personal statement as to why you want to be a dental hygienist or assistant.

Another way to find a position or at least a dental office that is open to curious students is to start with your high school guidance counselor or website. Also visit the websites listed in this book and search the web for dental offices in your area. Don't be afraid to pick up the phone and call them. Be prepared to start by cleaning facilities, assisting staff with clerical work, and other such tasks. Being on-site, no matter what you're doing, will teach you more than you know. With a great attitude and work ethic, you will likely be given more responsibility over time.

> "I definitely recommend that anyone interested shadow a hygienist. Most dental offices are open to that and it will help you see if you like it. You'll see what they do and see the flow."—Adrienne Collins, dental hygienist

Once you are in your program, you will get many hours of hands-on experience as well.

GETTING EXPERIENCE IN THE DENTAL LAB TECHNICIAN FIELD

If you're currently in high school and you're seriously thinking about becoming a dental lab technician, the quickest and easiest way to find a lab near you is to reach out to your own dentist and ask who they use. Or you can ask a family friend who runs or works in a dental office. A Google search for "dental lab near me" will yield some pretty accurate results as well. If you live in a sizable urban area, you'll get a good list to start with. Don't be afraid to pick up the phone and call them.

Reach out with your career aspirations and start by asking good questions. The point is to show your curiosity. Ask to shadow a technician, remembering the guidelines about courtesy above. Don't expect to be paid for any of this effort at first. The benefit of volunteering is that it's much easier to get your foot in the door, but the drawback is that you typically will not be paid. However, with time and hard work, your volunteer position may turn into something else.

Look at these kinds of experiences as ways to learn about the profession, show people how capable you are, and make connections to others that could last your career. It may even help you to get into the lab of your choice, and it will definitely help you write your personal statement as to why you want to be a dental lab technician.

As mentioned, be prepared to start with small jobs and clerical tasks. With a good attitude and work ethic, you will be given more responsibility over time.

Tip: Don't forget that your high school guidance counselor can be a great source of information and connections as well.

Networking

Because it's so important, another last word about networking. It's important to develop mentor relationships even at this stage. Remember that about 85 percent of jobs are found through personal contacts. If you know someone in the field, don't hesitate to reach out. Be patient and polite, but ask for help, perspective, and guidance.

"A lot of jobs are word of mouth and just connecting with people you know. It helps a lot if you know someone, rather than just send a résumé into an office cold."
—Lindsey Jones, dental hygienist

If you don't know anyone, ask your school guidance counselor to help you make connections. Or pick up the phone yourself. Reaching out with a genuine interest in knowledge and a real curiosity about the field will go a long way. You don't need a job or an internship just yet—just a connection that could blossom into a mentoring relationship. Follow these important but simple rules for the best results when networking:

- Do your homework about a potential contact, connection, university, or employer before you make contact. Be sure to have a general understanding of what they do and why. But don't be a know-it-all. Be open and ready to ask good questions.
- Be considerate of professionals' time and resources. Think about what they can get from you in return for mentoring or helping you.
- Speak and write with proper English. Proofread all your letters, e-mails, and even texts. Think about how you will be perceived at all times.
- Always stay positive.

Summary

In this chapter, you learned even more about the three different careers in the dental health umbrella—dental assistant, dental hygienist, and dental laboratory technician. You've learned all about the educational requirements of these different fields, from college degrees to certificates after high school. You also learned about getting experience in these fields before you enter school as well as during the educational process. At this time, you should have a good idea of the educational requirements of each position. You hopefully even contemplated some questions about what kind of educational career path fits your strengths, time requirements, and wallet. Are you starting to picture your career plan? If not, that's okay, as there's still time.

Remember that no matter which of these professions you pursue, you must maintain current certifications and meet the continuing education requirements. This is very important in all health careers. Advances in understanding in the fields of dental health, medicine, nutrition, and more are continuous, and it's vitally important that you keep apprised of what's happening in your field. The bottom line is that you need to have a lifelong love of learning to succeed in any health career.

In chapter 3, we go into a lot more detail about pursing the best educational path. The chapter covers the best schools for what you want to do, as well as how to find the best value for your education. The chapter includes discussion about financial aid and scholarships. At the end of chapter 3, you should have a much clearer view of the educational landscape and how and where you fit in.

3

Pursuing the Education Path

*W*hen it comes time to start looking at colleges, universities, or postsecondary schools, many high schoolers tend to freeze up at the enormity of the job ahead of them. This chapter will help break down this process for you so it won't seem so daunting.

Yes, finding the right college or learning institution is an important one, and it's a big step toward achieving your career goals and dreams. The last chapter covered the various educational requirements of these professions, which means you should now be ready to find the right institution of learning. This isn't always just a process of finding the very best school that you can afford and can be accepted into, although that might end up being your path. It should also be about finding the right fit so that you can have the best possible experience during your post–high school years.

So here's the truth of it all—attending postsecondary schooling isn't just about getting a degree. It's about learning how to be an adult, managing your life and your responsibilities, being exposed to new experiences, growing as a person, and otherwise moving toward becoming an adult who contributes to society. College offers you an opportunity to actually become an interesting person with perspective on the world and empathy and consideration for people other than yourself, if you let it.

An important component of how successful college will be for you is finding the right fit, the right school that brings out the best in you and challenges you at different levels. I know, no pressure, right? Just as with finding the right profession, your ultimate goal should be to match your personal interests/goals/personality with the college's goals and perspective. For example, small liberal arts colleges have a much different "feel" and philosophy than Big 10 state schools. And rest assured that all this advice applies even when you're planning on attending community college or another postsecondary school.

Don't worry, though, in addition to these "soft skills," this chapter does dive into the nitty-gritty of finding the best schools, no matter what you want to do. In the dental health fields specifically, attending an accredited program is critical to future success, and we cover that in detail in this chapter.

Finding a School That Fits Your Personality

Before we get into the details of good schools for each profession, it will behoove you to take some time to consider what "type" of school will be best for you. If nothing else, answering questions like the following ones can help you narrow your search and focus on a smaller sampling of choices. Write your answers to these questions down somewhere where you can refer to them often, such as in your notes app on your phone:

- *Size:* Does the size of the school matter to you? Colleges and universities range from sizes of 500 or fewer students to 25,000 students.
- *Community location:* Would you prefer to be in a rural area, a small town, a suburban area, or a large city? How important is the location of the school in the larger world to you?
- *Distance from home:* How far away from home do you want/are you willing to go? Phrase this in terms of hours away or miles away.
- *Housing options:* What kind of housing would you prefer? Dorms, off-campus apartments, and private homes are all common options.
- *Student body:* How would you like the student body to "look"? Think about coed versus all-male and all-female settings, as well as the makeup of minorities, how many students are part-time versus full-time, and the percentage of commuter students.
- *Academic environment:* Consider which majors are offered and at which levels of degree. Research the student-faculty ratio. Are the classes taught often by actual professors or more often by the teaching assistants? Find out how many internships the school typically provides to students. Are independent study or study abroad programs available in your area of interest?

- *Financial aid availability/cost:* Does the school provide ample opportunities for scholarships, grants, work-study programs, and the like? Does cost play a role in your options (for most people, it does)?
- *Support services:* Investigate the strength of the academic and career placement counseling services of the school.
- *Social activities and athletics:* Does the school offer clubs that you are interested in? Which sports are offered? Are scholarships available?
- *Specialize programs:* Does the school offer honors programs or programs for veterans or students with disabilities or special needs?

Not all of these questions are going to be important to you and that's fine. Be sure to make note of aspects that don't matter so much to you, too, such as size or location. You might change your mind as you go to visit colleges, but it's important to make note of where you're at to begin with.

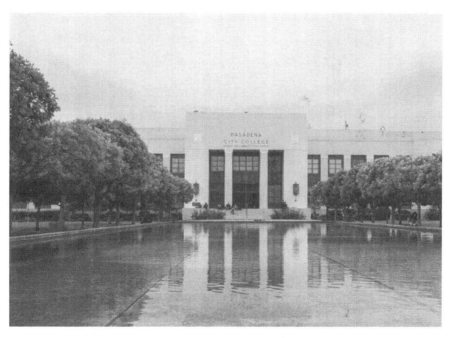

Community colleges, as long as they are accredited, can be great places of learning for a fraction of the cost.

U.S. News & World Report puts it best when they say the college that fits you best is one that will do all these things:

- Offers a degree that matches your interests and needs
- Provides a style of instruction that matches the way you like to learn
- Provides a level of academic rigor to match your aptitude and preparation
- Offers a community that feels like home to you
- Values you for what you do well

Note: According to the National Center for Educational Statistics (NCES), which is part of the US Department of Education, six years after entering college for an undergraduate degree, only 59 percent of students have graduated.[1] Barely half of those students will graduate from college in their lifetime.[2]

Hopefully, this section has impressed upon you the importance of finding the right college fit. Take some time to paint a mental picture about the kind of university or school setting that will best complement your needs. Then read on for specifics about each degree.

HOW IMPORTANT IS ACCREDITATION?

Keep in mind that many companies will only hire people who received their degrees from a program that has a specific accreditation. This is especially true in the health-related fields such as dentistry, which are more heavily regulated. When you research a school or program, make sure you can verify that the program of study is accredited through the proper accreditation body (which typically will be CODA). As we've discussed in previous chapters, some credentials are granted through state agencies and some are national boards, so you need to do a little research on your area of interest.

For more information on accreditation programs in general, visit these sites:[3]

- The Commission on Dental Accreditation (CODA) at www.ada.org/en/coda: This is part of the American Dental Association (ADA) and is charged with developing and implementing accreditation standards for dental education programs.

- The Accrediting Bureau of Health Education Schools at www.abhes.org: This accrediting agency is recognized by the US Department of Education and by the Council for Higher Education Accreditation.
- Commission on Accreditation of Allied Health Education Programs at www.caahep.org: Claims to be the largest programmatic accreditor in the health sciences field.

Your Degree Plan for Studies in Dental Health

If you're currently in high school and you are serious about pursuing a degree in dental health, whether it's as a dental hygienist, dental assistant, or dental lab technician, start by finding four to five schools in a realistic location (for you) that offer the degree/certificate/program in question. Not every school near you or that you have an initial interest in will probably offer the program you want of course, so narrow your choices accordingly. With that said, consider attending a university in your resident state, if possible, which will save you lots of money if you attend a state school. Private institutions don't typically discount resident student tuition costs.

Be sure you research the basic GPA and SAT or ACT requirements of each school as well.

Note: For those of you applying to associate's degree programs or greater, most advisors recommend that students take both the ACT and the SAT tests during their junior year (spring at the latest). (The ACT test is generally considered more weighted in science, so it may be more important when you're applying to dental health-type programs.) You can retake these tests and use your highest score, so be sure to leave time to retake early senior year if needed. You want your best score to be available to all the schools you're applying to by January of your senior year, which will also enable them to be considered with any scholarship applications. Keep in mind these are general timelines—be sure to check the exact deadlines and calendars of the schools to which you're applying!

Once you have found four to five schools in a realistic location for you that offer the degree/certificate in question, spend some time on their websites studying the requirements for admissions. Most universities will list the average stats for the last class accepted to the program. Important factors weighing on your decision of what schools to apply to should include whether or not you meet the requirements, your chances of getting in (but shoot high!), tuition costs and availability of scholarships and grants, location, and the school's reputation and licensure/graduation rates.

The order of these characteristics will depend on your grades and test scores, your financial resources, and other personal factors. You of course want to find a university that has a good reputation for the science and health fields, but it's also important to match your academic rigor and practical needs with the best school you can.

THE MOST PERSONAL OF PERSONAL STATEMENTS

The personal statement you include with your application to college is extremely important, especially when your GPA and SAT/ACT scores are on the border of what is typically accepted. Write something that is thoughtful and conveys your understanding of the profession you are interested in, as well as your desire to practice in this field. Why are you uniquely qualified? Why are you a good fit for this university? These essays should be highly personal (the "personal" in personal statement). Will the admissions professionals who read it, along with hundreds of others, come away with a snapshot of who you really are and what you are passionate about?

Look online for some examples of good ones, which will give you a feel for what works. Be sure to check your specific school for length guidelines, format requirements, and any other guidelines they expect you to follow.

And of course, be sure to proofread it several times and ask a professional (such as your school writing center or your local library services) to proofread it as well.

What's It Going to Cost You?

So, the bottom line—what will your education end up costing you? Of course that depends on many factors, including the type and length of degree, where you attend (in-state or not, private or public institution), how much in scholarships or financial aid you're able to obtain, your family or personal income, and many other factors. The College Entrance Examination Board (see www .collegeboard.org) tracks and summarizes financial data from colleges and universities all over the United States. A sample of the most recent data is shown in the following table.

Table 3.1. Average Yearly Tuition, Fees, Room and Board for Full-Time Undergraduates

Year	Public 2-Year	Public 4-Year, In-State	Public 4-Year, Out-of-State	Private Nonprofit
2016–2017	$11,640	$20,150	$35,300	$45,370
2017–2018	$11,970	$20,770	$36,420	$46,950

Source: College Entrance Examination Board website, www.collegeboard.org.

Keep in mind these are averages and reflect the published prices, not the net prices (see the following tip). If you read more specific data about a particular university or find averages in your particular area of interest, you should assume those numbers are closer to reality than these averages, as they are more specific. This data helps to show you the ballpark figures.

Another way to look at it is that completion of an associate's degree (two years) costs about $25,000–$30,000. You can expect to pay about half that for a one-year nondegree certificate.

Generally speaking, there is about a 3 percent annual increase in tuition and associated costs to attend college. In other words, if you are expecting to

---

Tip: The actual, final price (or "net price") that you'll pay for a specific college is the difference between the published price (tuition and fees) to attend that college, minus any grants, scholarships, and education tax benefits you receive. This difference can be significant. In 2015–2016, the average published price of in-state tuition and fees for public four-year colleges was about $9,410. But the average net price of in-state tuition and fees for public four-year colleges was only about $3,980.[4]

attend college two years after this data was collected, you need to add approximately 6 percent to these numbers. Keep in mind this assumes no financial aid or scholarships of any kind.

This chapter also covers finding the most affordable path to get the degree you want. Later in this chapter, you'll also learn how to prime the pumps and get as much money for college as you can.

WHAT IS A GAP YEAR?

Taking a year off between high school and college, often called a *gap year*, is normal, perfectly acceptable, and almost required in many countries around the world, and it is becoming increasingly acceptable in the United States as well. Even Malia Obama, President Obama's daughter, did it. Because the cost of college has gone up dramatically, it literally pays for you to know going in what you want to study, and a gap year—well spent—can do lots to help you answer that question.

Some great ways to spend your gap year include joining the Peace Corps or AmeriCorps organizations, enrolling in a mountaineering program or other gap year-styled program, backpacking across Europe or other countries on the cheap (be safe and bring a friend), find a volunteer organization that furthers a cause you believe in or that complements your career aspirations, join a Road Scholar program (see www.roadscholar.org), teach English in another country (see www.gooverseas.com/blog/best-countries-for-seniors-to-teach-english-abroad for more information), or work and earn money for college!

Many students will find that they get much more out of college when they have a year to mature and to experience the real world. The American Gap Year Association reports from their alumni surveys that students who take gap years show improved civic engagement, improved college graduation rates, and improved GPAs in college.[5]

See their website at gapyearassociation.org for lots of advice and resources if you're considering a potentially life-altering experience.

Your Dental Assistant Degree Plan

As you learned a little in the last chapter, many states have no training, credentialing, or continued education standards for dental assistants. Therefore, some dental assistants don't initially pursue any kind of postsecondary education before they begin working in the field. They learn mainly on the job, and then get certification in specialty areas (such as radiography and CPR training) as needed, while employed. In many states, this is certainly an option and the quickest way to begin earning a living while learning your trade, but it may be harder to break into this profession and find a job without any experience, unless you have personal connections or a little bit of luck and perseverance.

The other more sure-fire way to plan a career as a dental assistant is to attend an accredited program and receive certification. These programs usually take about one year to complete, after which you receive a certificate or diploma. Also, many states do require training for dental assistants, and a few states—including Minnesota, California, and Michigan—have even more specific educational standards and examinations for their registered dental assistants.[6]

> **Note:** The DALE Foundation maintains information on state requirements compiled by state dental boards. See www.dalefoundation.org/Resources-And-State-Requirements/State-Dental-Assistant-Requirements to determine exactly what's required in your state. This site also lists continuing education requirements by state as well.

Regardless of your state's requirements, becoming certified as a dental assistant shows potential employers that you are capable of performing the duties required. Many places of employment might require certification in order to be considered for a job even if your state does not.

CODA, part of the ADA, accredited nearly 300 dental assisting training programs in 2017. Most programs are offered through community colleges, although you can also find accredited programs through vocational or technical schools. The following image is from www.ada.org/en/coda, and shows the searchable listing of accredited schools. Although there are many ways to find schools on the Internet, it's best to start with this site so that you know you are looking at accredited programs.

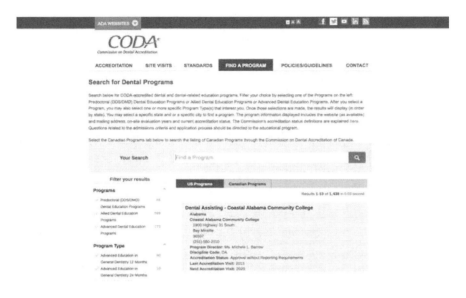

The CODA website lists only schools with proper accreditation.

There are also programs that last two years and lead to an associate's degree, but they are not as common. An associate's degree could make you more marketable in the long run, especially if you think you may work in different states or might want to become a dental hygienist at a later point, but of course they cost more in terms of time and money.

An accredited dental assistant program includes classroom and laboratory work. You will learn hands-on about teeth and gums, as well as other areas that dentists work on and the instruments that dentists use. These programs also include supervised practical experience.

STATISTICAL DATA

Recall that the average pay for a dental assistant in 2017 (the most recent data at the time of this writing) was $37,630. The job growth/outlook for the decade of 2016–2026 is 19 percent, which is faster than average. Being certified/licensed will better your job prospects as well.

Your Dental Hygienist Degree Plan

As discussed in the last chapter, you need an associate's degree from an accredited program in dental hygiene in order to practice as a dental hygienist. All states also require dental hygienists to be licensed.

Although the associate's degree is the most common path, there are also bachelor's and even master's degree programs in dental hygiene. You'll typically need a bachelor's or master's degree if you want to get into research, teaching, or clinical practice at public or school health programs. Whereas an associate's degree takes about two years, a bachelor's degree is usually a four-year commitment and a master's degree is another two years after that.

You will find that dental hygiene programs are typically offered by community colleges, technical schools, and universities. Your main resource for accredited schools, just as with the dental assistant career, is CODA. In 2017, CODA accredited more than 300 dental hygiene programs. See www.ada.org/en/coda for a fully searchable listing of accredited schools in your area.

Note: Keep in mind that community colleges and technical schools can be a much cheaper way (as much as half the cost) to attain the same degree, and as long as those programs are accredited by CODA, it won't matter to potential employers that you didn't attend a more well-known university.

The typical accredited dental hygiene program includes classroom, laboratory, and clinical work. Areas of study include physiology, nutrition, radiography, pathology, medical ethics, anatomy, patient management, and periodontics (the study of gum disease). You can prepare yourself in high school by loading up with classes like biology and anatomy.

LICENSING AND BOARD EXAMS

Although you are required to be licensed to practice as a dental hygienist, the requirements are determined by the states and so they vary across the United States. In nearly every state, you need to complete the following steps before you can apply for a dental hygienist license:

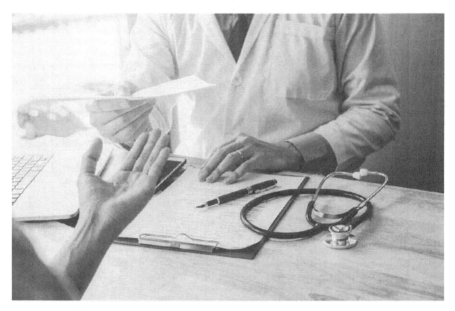

Getting certified and licensed as a dental hygienist takes several steps.

- Graduate from an accredited dental hygiene program.
- Pass the written National Board Dental Hygiene Examination (NDBHE).
- Pass a regional or state clinical board examination, depending on your state's requirements, to get your license.

Your best bet is to contact the licensing authority in your state for the specifics, although your postsecondary school or program should also have the most up-to-date information about those requirements. To maintain licensure, you also will have to complete continuing education requirements after you begin practicing.

Note: For the specific requirements in your state, check out www.dentalcareersedu .org/how-to-become-a-dental-hygienist. It includes a clickable map that provides detailed information about each state's exams and requirements to practice as a dental hygienist.

For lots more information about the licensing and examination process for dental hygienists, see chapter 2.

STATISTICAL DATA

The average pay for a dental hygienist in 2017 (the most recent data at the time of this writing) was $74,070. The job growth/outlook for the decade of 2016–2026 is 20 percent, which is much faster than the average.

MAKE THE MOST OF SCHOOL VISITS

If it's at all practical and feasible, you should visit the schools you're considering. To get a real feel for any college or school, you need to walk around the campus and buildings, spend some time in the common areas where students hang out, and sit in on a few classes. You can also sign up for campus tours, which are typically given by current students. This is another good way to see the school and ask questions of someone who knows. Be sure to visit the specific school/building that covers your possible major as well. The website and brochures won't be able to convey that intangible feeling you'll get from a visit.

In addition to the questions listed in the previous section in this chapter entitled "Finding a College That Fits Your Personality," consider these questions as well. Make a list of questions that are important to you before you visit.

- What is the makeup of the current freshman class? Is the campus diverse?
- What is the meal plan like? What are the food options?
- Where do most of the students hang out between classes? (Be sure to visit this area.)
- How long does it take to walk from one end of the campus to the other?
- What types of transportation are available for students? Does campus security provide escorts to cars, dorms, etc., at night?

In order to be ready for your visit and make the most of it, consider these tips and words of advice.

Before you go:
- Be sure to do some research. At the least, spend some time on the college website. Make sure your questions aren't addressed adequately there first.
- Make a list of questions.
- Arrange to meet with a professor in your area of interest or to visit the specific school.
- Be prepared to answer questions about yourself and why you are interested in this school.
- Dress in neat, clean, and casual clothes. Avoid overly wrinkled clothing or anything with stains.

During your visit:
- Listen and take notes.
- Don't interrupt.
- Be positive and energetic.
- Make eye contact when someone speaks directly to you.
- Ask questions.
- Thank people for their time.

Finally, be sure to send thank-you notes or e-mails after the visit is over. Remind the recipient when you visited the campus and thank them for their time.

Your Dental Lab Technician Degree Plan

As you learned in chapter 2, most dental laboratory technicians in the United States learn their trade from on-the-job training. Because all laboratories are different, the length of training varies.[7]

The good news is that a high school diploma, lots of persistence and luck, and maybe a personal connection, is usually enough to get an entry-level position as a dental laboratory technician. The trick is getting your foot in the door. Be sure to make the most of your high school years by taking courses in science, mathematics, computer programming, and art.

If you don't have a personal connection, start by finding all the dental appliance labs near where you live. This can be done with a simple search for "dental labs near me" on the Internet. If you start this process in high school, you might have an easier time selling yourself as an eager student/helper, especially if you're willing to be on cleanup or clerical duty in a volunteer position. It may not be exciting and it may not pay at first, but your foot is in the door. That's worth quite a lot. Show interest, curiosity, and a good attitude and work ethic, and any smart employer will keep you on and give you more responsibilities over time.

Before you reach out to any local lab, do research and know the basics— your state's regulations and requirements regarding dental lab techs, the basic terminology used in the industry (crown, implant, etc.—see the glossary of this book for more), corporate information about the lab you're looking at, and more. Be as educated as you can about the job you seek.

Although it's not required at this time, you can also pursue dental technician training through a two-year program at a community college, vocational school, technical college, university, or dental school. In most cases, you simply need a high school diploma or the equivalent to apply to an accredited dental laboratory technology program. The ADA has currently accredited more than 20 programs in dental laboratory technology from community colleges and other postsecondary schools (see www.ada.org for the most updated current list).

These training programs usually include courses in dental anatomy, dental ceramics, and dentures. You'll receive a short-term certificate or a two-year associate's degree from these programs, which is helpful to set you apart from others without these credentials.

Note: Be sure to take courses and gain experience in computer skills and programming. Dental appliances are more and more frequently being produced using highly advanced computer programs and three-dimensional printers.

Once you graduate from a program or are working as a dental lab technician, you can become a certified dental technician (CDT) by passing an examination that evaluates your technical skills and knowledge. Being certified can open advancement possibilities for you or help you get a raise. See the National Board for Certification in Dental Laboratory Technology (NBC) website at nbccert.org/homepage.cfm for current certification requirements.

STATISTICAL DATA

The average pay for a dental lab technician in 2017 (the most recent data at the time of this writing) was $35,250. The job growth/outlook for the decade of 2016–2026 is 13 percent, which is faster than the average.

BORN INTO DENTISTRY

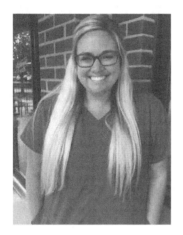

Adrienne Collins. *Courtesy of Adrienne Collins*

Adrienne Collins grew up around dentistry as her father is a dentist. She always found the dental world interesting as she hung around his office as a child. She received her dental hygienist certificate from Lakeland in Illinois and graduated in 2008 with an associate's degree in applied science. She has practiced for 10 years as a dental hygienist in Indiana and Illinois in general dentistry.

What is a typical day on your job?

We do chart preps in the morning for all the patients I will see that day. We see what services they are due for, any medical needs, and updates on health history. You do your cleanings with each patient, removing hard and soft deposits on the teeth. I also give X-rays and place fluoride and sealants when necessary, and take whitening impressions occasionally. I work along with the doctor to diagnose gum disease and evaluate the gums and teeth and mouth. The dentists come in to check the exams and answer questions from the patient. If there is a harder cleaning needed, hygienists can also administer a local anesthetic. I spend about 40 to 60 minutes with each patient and I see 8 to 12 patients a day.

What's the difference between corporate dentistry and working for a private dentist?

Dental corporations are large companies that manage a bunch of offices/satellites throughout the United States. They are run by a large organization and they hire dentists and hygienists to work in the offices.

I worked in corporate dentistry for several years because they provided me with health insurance. Once I got married and was eligible for my husband's health insurance, I decided to move to private practice because it suits me better. You get more time with each patient—the quality time with patients is better. You can get to know your patients better as well. The downfall is that private dentists don't usually offer health benefits to employees.

What's the best part of your job?

Helping patients! It's rewarding working with different patients and knowing that they feel better and that you are helping their overall health and oral health. Especially when they are fearful of the dentist and then they come in and say, "Oh my gosh, that wasn't too bad." They feel better.

What's the worst part of your job?

Not having health insurance as part of my job was a struggle. Also, the job can be repetitive and there isn't much variety. If you like a lot of change, it can get monotonous. The good thing is that you know what to expect.

Can you talk about the physicality of the job and how you combat any issues that come up?

I have definitely found myself having shoulder issues and carpal tunnel issues. In fact, a lot of hygienists leave the profession or clinicals because of these issues. Sometimes people don't last long in the field because of this. Because of the physicality of the job, 32 hours per week is considered full time and that's enough. Be sure to stretch and move positions throughout the day. Learning and practicing good posture is really important for your back and neck. Also, invest in *loupes*, which are microscopic glasses especially fitted for you. They help you to not have to bend over or be in unnatural positions so much. They are expensive but well worth it.

What's the most surprising thing about your job?

Finding a full-time job was harder than I thought it would be. The market was hard at first in Illinois and Indiana. Full- and part-time are both available, but it's much easier to find a part-time job, at least from my experience. Many hygienists work at a few different offices to get a full week's work.

What's next, where do you see yourself going from here?
I see myself continuing with this career for a long time. At some point, I might like to get into dental sales or teaching. The job is strenuous on your body so I might not do it forever.

Did your education prepare you for the job?
As far as cleaning and the hands-on stuff it did, but not as far as the insurance aspect and the computer software knowledge I needed. Once you get out, there is a much broader range of patients and people, which you don't really see in school as much. It takes practice to adapt and work with each type of personality out there.

Is it different now than it was with your dad's practice?
It has changed. Insurance dictates a lot of treatment and that can be tough because it's not always best for patients or they have to pay out of pocket. Some offices can focus more on sales by trying to sell extra things to make the office money.

What would be your advice to a young person who is considering becoming a dental hygienist?
If you like things to be consistent, it's good. It's rewarding helping people. If you aren't a big fan of blood, it's probably not for you. Be prepared to study a lot because it's not always easy. I definitely recommend shadowing a hygienist office; most offices are open to that and it will help you see if you like it. You can see what they do and see the flow.

Every office and every doctor is different, so keep that in mind. As a dental hygienist, you can work clinically, for a school, or in sales, so there are options. Talk to other hygienists to get their opinions.

Financial Aid and Student Loans

Finding the money to attend college, whether it is two or four years, an online program, or a vocational career college, can seem overwhelming. But you can do it if you have a plan before you actually start applying to college. If you get into your top-choice university, don't let the sticker cost turn you away. Financial aid can come from many different sources and it's available to cover all different kinds of costs you'll encounter during your years in college, including tuition, fees, books, housing, and food.

The good news is that universities more often offer incentive or tuition discount aid to encourage students to attend. The market is often more competitive in the favor of the student and colleges and universities are responding by offering more generous aid packages to a wider range of students than they used to. Here are some basic tips and pointers about the financial aid process:

- You apply for financial aid during your senior year. You must fill out the FAFSA (Free Application for Federal Student Aid) form, which can be filed starting October 1 of your senior year until June of the year you graduate.[8] Because the amount of available aid is limited, it's best to apply as soon as you possibly can. See fafsa.gov to get started.

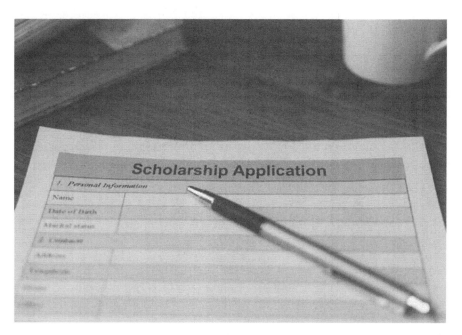

Paying for college can take a creative mix of grants, scholarships, and loans, but you can find your way with some help!

- Be sure to compare and contrast deals you get at different schools. There is room to negotiate with universities. The first offer for aid may not be the best you'll get.
- Wait until you receive all offers from your top schools and then use this information to negotiate with your top choice to see if they will match or beat the best aid package you received.
- To be eligible to keep and maintain your financial aid package, you must meet certain grade/GPA requirements. Be sure you are very clear on these academic expectations and keep up with them.
- You must reapply for federal aid every year.

Note: Watch out for scholarship scams! You should never be asked to pay to submit the FAFSA form ("free" is in its name) or be required to pay a lot to find appropriate aid and scholarships. These are free services. If an organization promises you you'll get aid or that you have to "act now or miss out," these are both warning signs of a less reputable organization.

Also, be careful with your personal information to avoid identity theft as well. Simple things like closing and exiting your browser after visiting sites where you entered personal information (like fafsa.gov) goes a long way. Don't share your student aid ID number with anyone either.

It's important to understand the different forms of financial aid that are available to you. That way, you'll know how to apply for different kinds and get the best financial aid package that fits your needs and strengths. The two main categories that financial aid falls under is gift aid, which don't have to be repaid, and self-help aid, which are either loans that must be repaid or work-study funds that are earned. The next sections cover the various types of financial aid that fit in one of these areas.

GRANTS

Grants typically are awarded to students who have financial needs, but can also be used in the areas of athletics, academics, demographics, veteran support, and special talents. They do not have to be paid back. Grants can come from federal agencies, state agencies, specific universities, and private organizations. Most federal and state grants are based on financial need.

Examples of grants are the Pell Grant, SMART Grant, and the Federal Supplemental Educational Opportunity Grant (FSEOG). Visit the US Department of Education's Federal Student Aid site for lots of current information about grants (see studentaid.ed.gov/types/grants-scholarships).

There have also been federal grants for healthcare professionals who are willing to work in less-served areas, and this has been true for dental health professionals too. If you're willing to work in states or communities that have been traditionally underserved with dental services (including Indian reservations), you can receive federal grants and benefits.

SCHOLARSHIPS

Scholarships are merit-based aid that does not have to be paid back. They are typically awarded based on academic excellence or some other special talent, such a music or art. Scholarships also fall under the areas of athletic-based, minority-based, aid for women, and so forth. These are typically not awarded by federal or state governments, but instead come from the specific school you applied to as well as private and nonprofit organizations.

Be sure to reach out directly to the financial aid officers of the schools you want to attend. These people are great contacts that can lead you to many more sources of scholarships and financial aid. Visit www.gocollege.com/financial-aid/scholarships/types for lots more information about how scholarships in general work.

LOANS

Many types of loans are available especially to students to pay for their post-secondary education. However, the important thing to remember here is that loans must be paid back, with interest. Be sure you understand the interest rate you will be charged. This is the extra cost of borrowing the money and is usually a percentage of the amount you borrow. Is this fixed or will it change over time? Is the loan and interest deferred until you graduate (meaning you don't have to begin paying it off until after you graduate)? Is the loan subsidized (meaning the federal government pays the interest until you graduate)? These are all points you need to be clear about before you sign on the dotted line.

There are many types of loans offered to students, including need-based loans, non-need-based loans, state loans, and private loans. Two very reputable federal loans are the Perkins Loan and the Direct Stafford Loan. For more information about student loans, start at bigfuture.collegeboard.org/pay-for-college/loans/types-of-college-loans.

FEDERAL WORK-STUDY

The US federal work-study program provides part-time jobs for undergraduate and graduate students with financial need so they can earn money to pay for educational expenses. The focus of such work is on community service work and work related to a student's course of study. Not all schools participate in this program, so be sure to check with the school financial aid office if this is something you are counting on. The sooner you apply, the more likely you will get the job you desire and be able to benefit from the program, as funds are limited. See studentaid.ed.gov/sa/types/work-study for more information about this opportunity.

HELPING PEOPLE FEELS GOOD

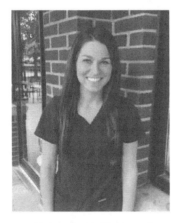

Lindsey Jones. *Courtesy of Lindsey Jones*

Lindsey Jones graduated in 2015 from the Indiana University School of Dentistry with a Bachelor's of Science in Public Health. She initially received her associate's degree, began working, and then pursued her bachelor's degree part-time, which took an additional year. She has worked as a dental hygienist in general practice dentistry since May 2015.

Explain the process you went through to find employment after you graduated?

I started off two days at one practice and subbed around on my other days, as it was difficult to find a full-time job at that time, especially when you don't have any experience. It helps to know someone, too. Hygienists who want full time often have to match up their days at different practices. I was able to work full-time, but at two different practices. I am now working full-time at only one private office and have been there about two and half years. My school even warned us that we might not find full-time work at first and you should take what you can get. Some people like the part-time aspect.

What is a typical day on your job?

It's mostly digital charts, and you go through and see what's needed for each patient, such as X-rays, what kind of cleaning they need, what kind of recall they are on, exam or not, and so on. Some offices do huddles in the morning. Some offices give you 30 minutes to prepare in the morning, whereas others ask you be there 15 minutes early to prepare in the morning. My standard jobs are cleanings, fluorides, X-rays, sealants, and educating the patient. Really, the whole thing is educating patients about oral health and hygiene so they can do a better job.

What's the best part of your job?

I like to help people feel better about themselves and be happier and healthier. I can give them easy tips to have better oral hygiene.

What's the worst part of your job?

I would say that it's the patients who don't want to be there and you have to try to win them over. That's easier said than done.

Can you talk about the physicality of the job and how you combat any issues that come up?

The physicality is a big issue. It's good to stretch throughout the day and keep fit and active. Back, neck, and shoulders are the problem areas.

My advice is to stretch and take very good care of yourself, or you can get burned out in this profession. Invest in loupes and use good chairs, saddle chairs. Overall the office layout makes a big difference in terms of if you're straining or not. Loupes you have to buy yourself because they are fitted especially for you.

What's the most surprising thing about your job?

Every office does things differently so you need to adapt to it or choose what you will be okay with. Some offices don't do things correctly. Some ethical practices I found surprising. Some offices are more production based and not as ethical. I prefer quality over quantity.

What's next, where do you see yourself going from here?

Eventually, I want to move to part time. I also want to move to sales (dental products) or education, which is why I got my bachelor's. Physically, I don't think it's something I could do full time forever.

Did your education prepare you for the job?

Yes, absolutely. Once you reach the second semester of hygiene school, you have classes and clinic every day. They prepared us very well. The patient pool at the IU School of Dentistry was very good. There was a certain amount of cleanings required—Class I–IV cleanings and Class IV is the hardest plaque—this all eases you into your boards. We even had mock boards. There are board review classes on the weekend to prepare as well.

Is the job what you expected?

It is, although I thought everything would be a little bit more standard, so you have to be ready to adjust yourself to different situations and work environment.

What would be your advice to a young person who is considering becoming a dental hygienist?

I took a career info class in high school and then shadowed my hygienist at my dentist's office. I got a lot of information from her, and that helped me out a lot. Then I did my own research. Definitely talk to a hygienist and visit a couple offices to see if you like the atmosphere. It helps you know if you can actually handle the job. I would recommend the profession. It's a good profession—you don't work weekends! Corporate dentistry is not as good, in my opinion. The scheduling is great.

Get all the information you can and talk to other hygienists. Get different opinions. Meet the doctors and see what they are like, too.

Making High School Count

If you are still in high school or middle school, there are still many things you can do now to help the postsecondary educational process go more smoothly. Consider these tips for your remaining years:

- Work on listening well and speaking and communicating clearly. Work on writing clearly and effectively.
- Learn how to learn. This means keeping an open mind, asking questions, asking for help when you need it, taking good notes, and doing your homework.
- Plan a daily homework schedule and keep up with it. Have a consistent, quiet place to study.
- Talk about your career interests with friends, family, and counselors. They may have connections to people in your community who you can shadow or will mentor you.
- Try new interests or activities, especially during your first two years of high school.
- Be involved in extracurricular activities that truly interest you and say something about who you are and want to be.

Kids are under so much pressure these days to "do it all," but you should think about working smarter rather than harder. If you are involved in things you enjoy, your educational load won't seem like such a burden. Be sure to take time for self-care, such as sleep, unscheduled down time, and other activities that you find fun and energizing. See chapter 4 for more ways to relieve and avoid stress.

Summary

This chapter dove right in and talked about all the aspects of college and postsecondary schooling that you'll want to consider as you move forward. Remember that finding the right fit is especially important, as it increases the chances that you'll stay in school and finish your degree or program, as well as have an amazing experience while you're there. The careers covered in this book have varying educational requirements, which means that finding the right school can be very different depending on your career aspirations.

In this chapter, you learned about the great schools out there and how to get the best education for the best deal. You also learned a little about scholarships and financial aid, how the SAT and ACT tests work, and how to write a unique personal statement that eloquently expresses your passions.

Use this chapter as a jumping off point to dig deeper into your particular area of interest. Some tidbits of wisdom to leave you with:

- If you need to, take the SAT and ACT tests early in your junior year so you have time to take them again. Most schools automatically accept the highest scores.
- Make sure that the school you plan to attend has an accredited program in your field of study. This is particularly important in the dental health field. Some professions follow national accreditation policies, while others are state-mandated and therefore differ across state lines. Do your research and understand the differences.
- Be sure the school or program you're looking at is CODA accredited. This is more important than any "big name" or high price tag.
- Don't underestimate how important school visits are, especially in the pursuit of finding the right academic fit. Come prepared to ask questions not addressed on the school website or in the literature.
- Your personal statement is a very important piece of your application that can set you apart from others. Take the time and energy needed to make it unique and compelling.
- Don't assume you can't afford a school based on the "sticker price." Many schools offer great scholarships and aid to qualified students. It doesn't hurt to apply. This advice especially applies to minorities, veterans, and students with disabilities.
- Don't lose sight of the fact that it's important to pursue a career that you enjoy, are good at, and are passionate about! You'll be a happier person if you do so.

At this point, your career goals and aspirations should be gelling. At the least, you should have a plan for finding out more information. And don't forget about networking, which was covered in more detail in chapter 2. Remember to do the research about the school or degree program before you reach out and especially before you visit. Faculty and staff find students who ask challenging questions much more impressive than those who ask questions that can be answered by spending 10 minutes on the school website.

In chapter 4, we go into detail about the next steps—writing a résumé and cover letter, interviewing well, follow-up communications, and more. This is information you can use to secure internships, volunteer positions, summer jobs, and more. It's not just for college grads. In fact, the sooner you can hone these communication skills, the better off you'll be in the professional world.

Writing Your Résumé and Interviewing

*N*o matter which path you decide to take—whether you enter the work-force immediately after high school, go to college first and then find yourself looking for a job, or maybe do something in between, having a well-written résumé and impeccable interviewing skills will help you reach your ultimate goals. This chapter provides some helpful tips and advice to build the best résumé and cover letter, how to interview well with all your prospective employers, and how to communicate effectively and professionally at all times. All the advice in this chapter isn't just for people entering the workforce full-time either. It can help you score that internship or summer job or help you give a great college interview to impress the admissions office.

After we talk about writing your résumé, the chapter discusses important interviewing skills that you can build and develop over time. The chapter also has some tips for dealing successfully with stress, which is an inevitable by-product of a busy life. Let's dive in!

Writing Your Résumé

If you're a teen writing a résumé for your first job, you likely don't have a lot of work experience under your belt yet. Because of this limited work experience, you need to include classes and coursework that are related to the job you're seeking, as well as any school activities and volunteer experience you have. While you are writing your résumé, you might discover some talents and recall some activities you did that you forgot about, which are still important to add. Think about volunteer work, side jobs you've held (baby sitting, dog walking, etc.), and the like. A good approach at this point in your career is to build a functional-type résumé, which focuses on your abilities rather than work expe-rience, and it's discussed in detail next.

PARTS OF A RÉSUMÉ

As mentioned, the functional résumé is the best approach when you don't have a lot of pertinent work experience, as it is written to highlight your abilities rather than the experience. The other, perhaps more common, type of résumé is called the chronological résumé and it lists a person's accomplishments in chronological order, most recent jobs listed first. This section breaks down and discusses the functional résumé in greater detail.

Here are the essential parts of your résumé, listed from the top down:

- *Heading*—This should include your name, address, and contact information, including phone, e-mail, and website if you have one. This information is typically centered on the page.
- *Objective*—This is one sentence that tells that specific employer what kind of position you are seeking. These should be modified to be specific to each potential employer.
- *Education*—Always list your most recent school or program first. Include date of completion (or expected date of graduation), degree or certificate earned, and the institution's name and address. Include workshops, seminars, and related classes here as well.
- *Skills*—Skills include computer literacy, leadership skills, organizational skills, or time-management skills. Be specific in this area when possible.
- *Activities*—These can be related to skills. Perhaps an activity listed here led to you developing a skill listed above. This section can be combined with the Skills section, but it's often helpful to break these apart if you have enough substantive things to say in both areas. Examples include sports teams, leadership roles, community service work, clubs and organizations, and so on.
- *Experience*—If you don't have any actual work experience that's relevant, you might consider skipping this section. However, you can list summer, part-time, and volunteer jobs you've held.
- *Interests*—This section is optional, but it's a chance to include special talents and interests. Keep it short, factual, and specific.
- *References*—It's best to say that references are available on request. If you do list actual contacts, list no more than three and make sure you inform your contacts that they might be contacted.

The first three entries above are pretty much standard, but the other entries can be creatively combined or developed to maximize your abilities and experience. These are not set-in-stone sections that every résumé must have. As an example, consider this mock functional résumé.

Piper Ellen Corcoran

974 Audubon Circle
Portland, OR, 97035
Phone: 503-503-5030 E-Mail: pec2001@student.com

Objective

Seeking an entry-level position to further my passion and desire to work in the dental health industry

Education

High School Diploma, June 2018
Westhaven High School, Portland, OR
GPA: 3.87. Top 4% of class

Skills

Computer literacy on PC and Mac; MS Word, Excel, PowerPoint, desktop publishing, web software
Trained in first aid and CPR
Four years of Spanish

Activities

Captain of the Spanish Club, 2018
Outstanding Community Service Award, 2017
Volunteer tutor of Spanish to ESL students, 2017-2018

Experience

2018 internship co-op participant, Standport Dental Care Facility, Portland OR
June 2016-June 2017, Part-time volunteer, Primelife Dental Health, Portland, OR
May 2015-June 2016, Crew Team Member, Big Burger Stop 'N Eat, Portland, OR

References

Available upon request

A functional-style résumé is a good template to use when you don't have a lot of work experience.

If you're still not seeing the big picture here, it's helpful to look at student and part-time résumé examples online to see how others have approached this process. Search for "functional résumé examples" to get a look at some examples.

RÉSUMÉ-WRITING TIPS

Regardless of your situation and why you're writing the résumé, there are some basic tips and techniques you should use:

- Keep it short and simple. This includes using a simple, standard font and format. Using one of the résumé templates provided by your word processor software can be a great way to start.
- Use simple language. Keep it to one page.
- Highlight your academic achievements, such as a high GPA (above 3.5) or academic awards. If you have taken classes related to the job you're interviewing for, list those briefly as well.
- Emphasize your extracurricular activities, internships, etc. These could include clubs, sports, dog walking, babysitting, or volunteer work. Use these activities to show your skills and abilities.
- Use action verbs, such as led, created, taught, ran, developed.
- Be specific and give examples.
- Always be honest.
- Include leadership roles and experience.
- Edit and proofread at least twice and have someone else do the same. Ask a professional (such as your school writing center or your local library services) to proofread it for you also. Don't forget to run spell check.
- Include a cover letter (discussed next).

THE COVER LETTER

Every résumé you send out should include a cover letter. This can be the most important part of your job search because it's often the first thing that potential employers read. By including the cover letter, you're showing the employers that you took the time to learn about their organization and address them personally. This goes a long way to show that you're interested in the position.

Be sure to call the company or verify on the website the name and title of the person to whom you should address the letter. This letter should be brief. Introduce yourself and begin with a statement that will grab the person's attention. Keep in mind that they will potentially be receiving hundreds of résumés and cover letters for an open position. You want yours to stand out. Important information to include in the cover letter, from the top, includes:

- The current date
- Your address and contact information
- The person's name, company, and contact information

Then you begin the letter portion of the cover letter, which should mention how you heard about the position, something extra about you that will interest the potential employer, practical skills you can bring to the position, and past experience related to the job. You should apply the facts outlined in your résumé to the job to which you're applying. Each cover letter should be personalized for the position/company to which you're applying. Don't use "to whom it may concern." Instead, take the time to find out to whom you should actually address the letter. Finally, end with a complimentary closing, such as "Sincerely, Henry Smith" and be sure to add your signature. Search for "sample cover letters for internships" or "sample cover letters for high schoolers" to see some good examples. As an example, consider this mock cover letter as an example.

Piper Ellen Corcoran
974 Audubon Circle
Portland, OR 97035

Ms. Sylvia Gonzalez
Director of Human Resources
City Dental
511 W 10th Ave.
Portland, OR 97035

Dear Ms. Gonzalez,

I'm writing based on the article I read in the October 9th edition of the *Portland Star*. In the article, you were quoted as saying "we need more skilled intake personnel to effectively serve the growing Spanish-speaking population" around your facility.

I believe my experience with both the Spanish language and with local dental care facilities can help address the need you have at City Dental. I have four years of Spanish experience, and I can speak near fluently. For the past two years, I've served as a part-time tutor for students who know English as a second language (ESL). This has helped me improve my Spanish and given me terrific interpersonal skills.

I'm ready to use my Spanish skills in the dental care environment, which is my career goal. I've had several internships and cooperative experiences in local dental care, including a co-op position at Standport Dental Care facility, where I worked with both patients and their families. I'm very good at understanding the needs of others and communicating them to healthcare workers. My computer experience will be a great help in the data entry required of every intake worker.

I'm eager to put my skills to work in your organization, because all parties will benefit from my experience. I look forward to hearing from you at your convenience.

Sincerely,

Piper E. Corcoran

Piper E. Corcoran

Your cover letter can be the most important part of your job search because it's often the first thing potential employers see.

If you are e-mailing your cover letter instead of printing it out, you'll need to pay particular attention to the subject line of your e-mail. Be sure that it is specific to the position you are applying for. In all cases, it's really important to follow the employer's instructions on how to submit your cover letter and résumé. Generally speaking, sending PDF documents rather than editable DOC forms is a better idea. For one, everyone can read a PDF, whereas they might not be able to read the version of Word, etc., that you used. Most word processing programs have an option under the Save command that allows you to save your work as a PDF.

EFFECTIVELY HANDLING STRESS

As you're forging ahead with you life plans, whether it's college, a full-time job, or even a gap year, you might find that these decisions feel very important and heavy and that the stress is difficult to deal with. First off, that's completely normal. Try these simple stress-relieving techniques:

- Take deep breaths in and out. Try this for 30 seconds. You'll be amazed at how it can help.
- Close your eyes and clear your mind.
- Go scream at the passing subway car. Or lock yourself in a closet and scream. Or scream into a pillow. For some people, this can really help.
- Keep the issue in perspective. Any decision you make now can be changed if it doesn't work out.

Want ways to avoid stress altogether? They are surprisingly simple. Of course, simple doesn't always mean easy, but it means they are basic and make sense with what we know about the human body:

- Get enough sleep
- Eat healthy
- Get exercise
- Go outside
- Schedule downtime
- Connect with friends and family

The bottom line is that you need to take time for self-care. There will always be conflict, but how you deal with it makes all the difference. This only becomes increasingly important as you enter college or the workforce and maybe have a family. Developing good, consistent habits related to self-care now will serve you all your life.

"Being a dental hygienist can take a toll on your body. It's a lot of repetitive motion. You are in positions that aren't great for your muscles and it can be hard on your shoulders, neck, back, and wrists. You need to take care of yourself. Exercise and stretching is important. Getting massages once a month is a good idea. It helps to loosen your muscles."—Catherine Kimmey, dental hygienist

Interviewing Skills

The best way to avoid nerves and keep calm when you're interviewing is to be prepared. It's okay to feel scared, but keep it in perspective. It's likely that you'll receive many more rejections in your professional life than acceptances, as we all do. However, you only need one "yes" to start out. Think of the interviewing process as a learning experience. With the right attitude, you will learn from each experience and get better each subsequent interview. That should be your overarching goal. Consider these tips and tricks when interviewing, whether it be for a job, internship, college admission, or something else entirely:[1]

- Practice interviewing with a friend or relative. Practicing will help calm your nerves and make you feel more prepared. Ask for specific feedback from your friends. Do you need to speak louder? Are you making enough eye contact? Are you actively listening when the other person is speaking?
- Learn as much as you can about the company, school, or organization. Also be sure to understand the position for which you're applying. This will show the interviewer that you are motivated and interested in their organization.
- Speak up during the interview. Convey to the interviewer important points about you. Don't be afraid to ask questions. Try to remember the interviewers names and call them by name.
- Arrive early and dress professionally and appropriately (you can read more about proper dress in a following section).
- Take some time to prepare answers to commonly asked questions. Be ready to describe your career or educational goals to the interviewer.

Common questions you may be asked during a job interview include these:

- Tell me about yourself.
- What are your greatest strengths?
- What are your weaknesses?
- Tell me something about yourself that's not on your résumé.
- What are your career goals?
- How do you handle failure? Are you willing to fail?
- How do you handle stress and pressure?
- What are you passionate about?
- Why do you want to work for us?

Common questions you may be asked during a college admissions interview include these:

- Tell me about yourself.
- Why are you interested in going to college?
- Why do you want to major in this subject?
- What are your academic strengths?
- What are your academic weaknesses? How have you addressed them?
- What will you contribute to this college/school/university?
- Where do you see yourself in ten years?
- How do you handle failure? Are you willing to fail?
- How do you handle stress and pressure?
- Whom do you most admire?
- What is your favorite book?
- What do you do for fun?
- Why are you interested in this college/school/university?

Jot down notes about your answers to these questions, but don't try to memorize the answers. You don't want to come off too rehearsed during the interview. Remember to be as specific and detailed as possible when answering these questions. Your goal is to set yourself apart in some way from the other people they will interview. Always accentuate the positive, even when you're asked about something you did not like, or about failure or stress. Most importantly, though, be yourself.

> **Tip:** Active listening is the process of fully concentrating on what is being said, understanding it, and providing nonverbal cues and responses to the person talking.[2] It's the opposite of being distracted and thinking about something else when someone is talking. Active listening takes practice. You might find that your mind wanders and you need to bring it back to the person talking (and this could happen multiple times during one conversation). Practice this technique in regular conversations with friends and relatives. In addition to giving a better interview, it can cut down on nerves and make you more popular with friends and family, as everyone wants to feel that they are really being heard. For more on active listening, check out www.mindtools.com/CommSkll/ActiveListening.htm.

You should also be ready to ask questions of your interviewer. In a practical sense, there should be some questions that you have that you can't find the answer to on the website or in the literature. Also, asking questions shows that you are interested and have done your homework. Avoid asking questions about salary/scholarships or special benefits at this stage, and don't ask about anything negative that you've heard about the company or school. Keep the questions positive and relative to you and the position to which you're applying. Some example questions to potential employers include:

- What is a typical career path for a person in this position?
- How would you describe the ideal candidate for this position?
- How is the department organized?
- What kind of responsibilities come with this job? (Don't ask this if they've already addressed this question in the job description or discussion.)
- What can I do as a follow-up?
- When do you expect to reach a decision?

See the section in chapter 3 entitled "Make the Most of Campus Visits" for some good example questions to ask the college admissions office. The important thing is to write your own questions related to answers you really want to know. This will show genuine interest. Be sure your question isn't answered on the website, in the job description, or in the literature.

Dressing Appropriately

It's important to determine what is actually appropriate in the setting of the interview. What is appropriate in a corporate setting might be different from what you'd expect as a small liberal arts college or at a large hospital setting. Most college admissions offices suggest "business casual" dress, for example, but depending on the job interview, you may want to step it up from there. Again, it's important to do your homework and come prepared. In addition to reading up on their guidelines, it never hurts to take a look around the site if you can to see what other people are wearing to work or to interviews. Regardless of the setting, make sure your clothes are not wrinkled, untidy, or stained. Avoid flashy clothing of any kind.

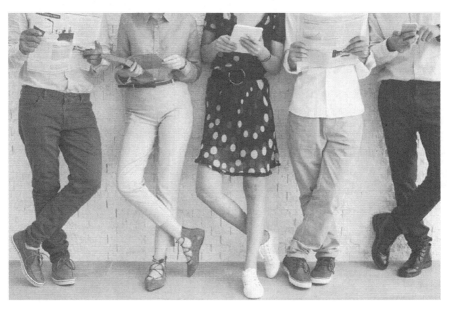

Even something like "business casual" can be interpreted in many ways, so do some research to find out what exactly is expected of you.

Follow-Up Communication

Be sure to follow up, whether in e-mail or via regular mail, with a thank-you note to the interviewer. This is true whether you're interviewing for a job or internship or interviewing with a college. A hand-written thank you note, posted in the actual mail, is best. In addition to being considerate, it will trigger the interviewer's memory about you and it shows that you have genuine interest in the position, company, or school. Be sure to follow the business-letter format and highlight the key points of your interview and experience at the company/university. And be prompt with your thank-you! Put it in the mail the day after your interview (or send that e-mail the same day).

What Employers Expect

Regardless of the job, profession, or field you end up working in, there are universal characteristics that all employers (and schools, for that matter) look for in potential employees. At this early stage in your professional life, you have an opportunity to recognize which of these foundational characteristics are your strengths (and therefore highlight them in an interview) and which are weaknesses (and therefore continue to work on them and build them up). Consider these universal characteristics that all employers look for:

- Positive attitude
- Dependability
- Desire to continue to learn
- Initiative
- Effective communication
- Cooperation
- Organization

This is not an exhaustive list, and other characteristics can very well include things like being sensitive to others, being honest, having good judgment, being loyal, being responsible, and being on time. Specifically in healthcare/dental care, you can add having empathy, being flexible, having good attention to detail, and being physically fit to that list. Consider these important characteristics when you answer the common questions that employers ask. It pays to work these traits into the answers, of course being honest and realistic about your traits.

Beware the social media trap! Prospective employers and colleges will check your social media sites, so make sure there is nothing too personal, explicit, or inappropriate on your sites. When you communicate out to the world in this way, don't use profanity and be sure to use proper grammar. Think about the version of yourself you are portraying online. Is it favorable or at least neutral to potential employers? They will look, rest assured.

A RETIRED DENTAL HYGIENIST SPEAKS OUT

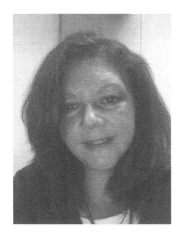

Julia Guy. *Courtesy of Julia Guy*

Julia Guy received her dental hygienist certificate from Howard University, Washington DC, in 1993. She practiced for 21 years as a dental hygienist, retiring due to neck and shoulder pain in 2014. She went back to school and got a bachelor's degree and is now doing financial management for the government. Despite leaving the career, she enjoyed it greatly and encourages anyone interested in doing it to pursue it.

Can you explain how you became interested in being a dental hygienist and the specific educational process you went through?

I was thinking about nursing, but a friend was a dental manager (and used to be a nurse) and she told me that the hours and money were better as a dental hygienist and the issues were confined to the mouth. There were no nights and weekends, the money was good, you only deal with certain parts of the body, and you are your own boss more or less. It sounded too good to be true! At that time, the demand for hygienists was very high. There was a waiting list to get into school and I got in. I absolutely loved it!

What was a typical day in your job?

The first thing in the morning we had our huddle to discuss the day's patients, such as who is getting X-rays, fluoride, etc., treatments outstanding, and so on, so we could flag the doctor.

In the practice that I worked at the majority of my years, at first it was just me and one other hygienist. Over time, it grew to 16 chairs. Eventually, I became the hygiene manager and we had six hygiene chairs. I was in charge of the schedule and made sure it ran smoothly as I was seeing patients. I had an amazing assistant who would inform me if we were getting off schedule and we would rearrange which hygienists would see the next patients, to ensure everything ran smoothly and that patients weren't waiting too long.

I also did hands-on cleaning, went over X-rays, talked about outstanding treatment, prepared the patient for the doctor so the doctor knew what was going on as far as the overall plan for this patient. This gave the doctors a segue into the patient.

We worked 8-hour shifts at first, then it grew and became 12-hour days—so you could choose six-hour shifts, from 6 to 12 or 12 to 6. You could schedule your own hours as long as it worked with the whole group. It was flexible and allowed me to take my son to school certain mornings and work around his schedule. I saw about six patients per day, 50-minute appointments.

What was the best part of your job?

Dealing with the patients—they became my friends and I really miss them. I still see some of them on the street and they will come up and hug me. Many patients became "mine" over time, because I built a rapport with them. I would write notes in their charts about their personal lives, and why they came back in. I would ask about the vacations I knew they were taking. I was alone with patients 40 to 50 minutes before the doctor came in, so you got to know them. One of my favorite things was to win a patient over. Initially, they are scared but then, at the end of the appointment, they are happy and say, "that wasn't too bad!" Then they come back every six months and are committed to getting cleanings.

I also liked the freedom. You work directly with patients, not much doctor standing over you. You get to manage your own schedule after a while.

What was the worst part of your job?

Because the doctors had a program in the county to treat children of need in the community under a certain age, we treated a lot of underprivileged kids whose parents who weren't educated and didn't realize their kids were in pain. They didn't know that soda caused tooth decay, for example. It was hard to see those children suffering and in pain with preventable issues. With all this technology out there, the lack of knowledge that some people still have is hard for me to understand.

Did your education prepare you for the job?

Absolutely—I don't think you could learn all this on the job . . . the dental anatomy, head and neck anatomy, and pharmacology would be very hard to learn on the job. The board test was very detailed and studied for a whole week. There was also a physical part where you also had to clean someone's teeth. You had to find the patient with a certain amount of tartar in their mouth.

Was the job what you expected?

Yes, pretty much. It's very satisfying to clean someone's teeth and see the end result.

Can you talk more about why you left the profession?

In the end, it was due to my repetitive stress injuries. My hand would freeze up and I couldn't hold on to the air/water syringe anymore. My doctor took X-rays and did some therapy and eventually said it would not likely get better and would get worse as I got older. He told me that I may never be able to hold my hand in that aspect again.

When I started, they didn't have the big balls to sit on and other therapy approaches to avoid repetitive stress injuries. I got those things, eventually, but it was toward the last part of my career. It's better now because of the ergonomic chairs and equipment and lights on your head so you don't have to bend over so much and hold things so much. The cleaners are better, too, because you don't have to be as forceful with your hand. This will help the younger generation stay in the game longer. Someone in the field a long time and looking for the next phase could also get their master's degree and teach the next generation.

What would be your advice to a young person who is considering becoming a dental hygienist?

Take all prerequisites first and get them out of the way before the actual program. That allows you to study more and be more prepared. Enjoy it! It's a great career for a young person. You make good money; you can take care of your kids; you don't have to work full time if you don't want to. I always encourage people who are interested—they need them especially in the Midwest, on Indian Reservations, and in small communities.

Personal contacts can make the difference! Don't be afraid to contact people you know. Personal connections can be a great way to find jobs and internship opportunities. Your high school teachers, your coaches and mentors, and your friends' parents are all examples of people who very well may know about jobs or internships that would suit you. Start asking several months before you hope to start a job or internship, because it will take some time to do research and arrange interviews. You can also use social media in your search. LinkedIn, for example, includes lots of searchable information on local companies. Follow and interact with people on social media to get their attention. Just remember to act professionally and communicate with proper grammar, just as you would in person.

Summary

Well, you made it to the end of this book! Hopefully, you have learned enough about the dental health field to start your journey, or to continue with your path. If you've reached the end and you feel like one of these careers is right for you, that's great news. Or, if you've figured out that this isn't the right field for you, that's good information to learn, too. For many of us, figuring out what we *don't* want to do and what we don't like is an important step in finding the right career.

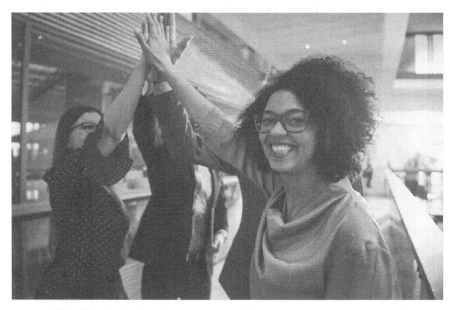

With a little hard work and perseverance, you'll be on your way to career success!

There is a lot of good news about the dental health field and it's a very smart career choice for anyone with a passion to help people. It's a great career for people who get energy from working with other people. Job demand is high and will continue to grow. Whether you decide to attend a four-year university, go to community college, or take a gap year, having a plan and an idea about your future can help guide your decisions. We hope that by reading this book, you are well on your way to having a plan for your future. Good luck to you as you move ahead!

Glossary

accreditation: The act of officially recognizing an organizational body, person, or educational facility as having a particular status or being qualified to perform a particular activity. For example, schools and colleges are accredited. *See also* certification.

ACT: The American College Test (ACT) is one of the standardized college entrance tests that anyone wanting to enter undergraduate studies in the United States should take. It measures knowledge and skills in mathematics, English, reading, and science reasoning, as they apply to college readiness. There are four multiple-choice sections. There is also an optional writing test. The total score of the ACT is 36. *See also* SAT.

active listening: The process of fully concentrating on what is being said, understanding it, and providing nonverbal cues and responses to the person talking. It's the opposite of being distracted and thinking about something else when someone is talking to you.

anatomy: The area of science concerned with the bodily structure and organization of humans, animals, and other living things.

associate's degree: A degree awarded by community or junior colleges that typically requires two years of study.

baby boomers: The American generation that was born after World War II, starting in about 1945, until about 1964. During this time, there was a "boom" (large increase) in the number of births in the United States. This matters to professionals in dental health because baby boomers continue to age and disproportionately need care and services that dental health professionals provide.

bachelor's degree: An undergraduate degree awarded by colleges and universities which is typically a four-year course of study when pursued full-time, but this can vary by degree earned and by the university awarding the degree.

calculus: Hardened dental plague deposits; another word for tartar. Caused by precipitation of minerals from saliva in plaque on the teeth.

cardiovascular system: The system of the human body making up the heart and blood, including veins and arteries. Applicable diseases include stroke, heart attack, and high blood pressure.

cementum: The calcified substance of a tooth found at the base that covers the root. One of the four major parts of a tooth, along with the enamel, dentin, and pulp.

certification: The action or process of confirming certain skills or knowledge on a person. Usually provided by some third-party review, assessment, or educational body. Individuals, not organizations, are certified. *See also* accreditation.

cosmetic dentistry: The area of dentistry that focuses on any dental work that improves the appearance (although not necessarily the functionality) of a patient's teeth.

dentin: The hard, dense tissue that makes up the bulk of a tooth, beneath the enamel. It's similar to but denser than bone. One of the four major parts of a tooth, along with the enamel, cementum, and pulp.

diagnosis: When a healthcare professional determines the nature of an illness or problem after examining a patient.

doctorate degree: The highest level of degree awarded by colleges and universities. Qualifies the holder to teach at the university level. Requires (usually published) research in the field. Typically requires an additional 3 to 5 years of study after earning a bachelor's degree. Anyone with a doctorate degree can be addressed as a "doctor," not just medical doctors.

enamel: The hardest and outermost substance of the tooth. It covers the outer layer of each tooth and is the most visible part of a tooth. One of the four major parts of a tooth, along with the dentin, cementum, and pulp.

endodontics: The study and treatment of the inside of the tooth, called the pulp. Most common procedure related to endodontics is a root canal treatment.

fluoride: Fluoride treatments make teeth more resistant to acid attacks from plaque, bacteria, and sugars in the saliva. These treatments prevent tooth decay and even can reverse early decay.

gap year: A gap year is a year between high school and college (or sometimes between college and postgraduate studies) whereby the student is not in school but is instead typically involved in volunteer programs, such as the Peace Corps, in travel experiences, or in work and teaching experiences.

grants: Money to pay for postsecondary education that is typically awarded to students who have financial needs, but can also be used in the areas of athletics, academics, demographics, veteran support, and special talents. Grants do not have to be paid back.

license: An official document, card, certificate, and so on, that gives you permission to have, use, or do something, such as practice as a dental hygienist. Typically, one gets certified and then applies for a license.

loupes: A simple small magnification device that is especially fitted for the user (dentist, dental hygienist, dental assistant, etc.) and attached to a glasses frame. They allow the user to focus on close-up work without straining their bodies.

master's degree: A secondary degree awarded by colleges and universities that requires at least one additional year of study after obtaining a bachelor's degree. The degree holder shows mastery of a specific field.

maxillofacial: A fancy word for the jaws and face.

oral and maxillofacial surgery: Removal of teeth and correction of facial deformities.

orthodontics and dentofacial orthopedics: Straightening teeth with braces or other appliances.

pathology: The science that identifies and manages diseases. In this case, diseases affecting the oral and maxillofacial areas.

pediatric dentistry: The branch of dentistry that studies and treats children exclusively.

periodontal probings: The process of using a tool to measure pocket depths around a tooth in order to establish the health of the tissues around the tooth.

periodontics: The study and treatment of the gums and bones supporting the teeth. These supporting tissues are known as the periodontium, which includes the gingiva, alveolar bone, cementum, and the periodontal ligament.

periodontics: The study of gum disease.

personal statement: A written description of your accomplishments, outlook, interest, goals, and personality that's an important part of your college application. The personal statement should set you apart from others. The required length depends on the institution, but they generally range from 1 to 2 pages, or 500 to 1,000 words.

plaque: A sticky clear, soft deposit that forms between teeth and above and below the gum line. Regular dental cleanings will remove plaque buildup.

postsecondary degree: Educational degree above and beyond a high school education. This is a general description that includes trade certificates and certifications, associate degrees, bachelor's degrees, master's degrees, and beyond.

prophylaxis: Any action taken to prevent disease. Oral prophylaxis would include mouth rinses, cleanings, and toothbrushing.

prosthodontics: The design, manufacture, and fitting of artificial replacements for teeth and other parts of the mouth (essentially, replacement of lost teeth).

pulp: The center of the tooth. It contains living connective tissue and cells. During a root canal process, the pulp of a diseased tooth is removed and replaced with dental filler. One of the four major parts of a tooth, along with the dentin, cementum, and enamel.

radiography: Imaging process that uses X-rays to view the internal structure of an opaque object—in this specific case, teeth and surrounding bones.

rehabilitation: The process of returning someone back to a healthier state, better health, or a more functional life after an illness or accident.

restorative dentistry: The area of dentistry that repairs damaged, diseased, or missing teeth and their supporting structures, in order to restore structure and function.

root planing: A deeper dental cleaning process that smoothens the tooth root and helps the gums reattach to the tooth.

SAT: The Scholastic Aptitude Test (SAT) is one of the standardized tests in the United States that anyone applying to undergraduate studies should take.

It measures verbal and mathematical reasoning abilities as they relate to predicting successful performance in college. It is intended to complement a student's GPA and school record in assessing readiness for college. The total score of the SAT is 1,600. *See also* ACT.

scaling: A deeper dental cleaning process that removes excessive plaque buildup from below the gum line and helps combat gum disease and restore dental health.

scholarships: Merit-based aid used to pay for postsecondary education that does not have to be paid back. Scholarships are typically awarded based on academic excellence or some other special talent, such as music or art.

sealant: A material placed in the pits and fissures in a tooth to fill them in, in order to prevent tooth decay. This creates a smooth surface that's easier to clean and less prone to plaque buildup. Dental sealants are mainly used in children who are at higher risk of tooth decay, and are usually placed as soon as the adult molar teeth come through.

tartar: Another word for calculus. *See also* calculus.

veneer: A thin layer placed over a tooth so as to improve the look of a tooth or to protect the tooth's surface.

Notes

Chapter 1

1. Adapted from American Dental Association, "Dental Assistant," www.ada
.org/en/education-careers/careers-in-dentistry/dental-team-careers/dental-assistant.

2. ADA.org/education-careers.

3. Adapted from American Dental Education Association, "History of Dentistry,"
www.adea.org/GoDental/Health_Professions_Advisors/History_of_Dentistry.aspx.

4. Adapted from Bureau of Labor Statistics, US Department of Labor, "Dental
Assistants," www.bls.gov/ooh/healthcare/dental-assistants.htm.

5. Adapted from American Dental Association, "Dental Hygenist," www.ada
.org/en/education-careers/careers-in-dentistry/dental-team-careers/dental-hygienist.

6. American Dental Association, "Careers in Dentistry," www.ada.org/en/educa
tion-careers/careers-in-dentistry.

7. Evan Andrews, "Did George Washington Have Wooden Teeth?" History.com,
April 30, 2014, www.history.com/news/did-george-washington-have-wooden-teeth.

8. Bureau of Labor Statistics, US Department of Labor, "Dental Hygenists,"
www.bls.gov/ooh/healthcare/dental-hygienists.htm.

9. American Dental Association, "Careers in Dentistry."

10. Bureau of Labor Statistics, US Department of Education, "Dental and
Ophthalmic Laboratory Technicians and Medical Appliance Technicians," www.bls.gov/
ooh/production/dental-and-ophthalmic-laboratory-technicians-and-medical-appli
ance-technicians.htm

Chapter 2

1. DentalHealthCareersEDU.org, "Becoming a Dental Hygenist or Dental
Assistant," www.dentalcareersedu.org.

2. DentalHealthCareersEDU.org, "Dental Assistant Requirements for State
Licensure and Registration," www.dentalcareersedu.org/dental-assistant-requirements
-for-state-licensure.

3. Virtual Career Network, "Dental Laboratory Technician," www.vcn.org/health-care/careers/51-9081.00/education-training.

4. See LinkedIn.com, "New Survey Reveals 85% of All Jobs Are Filled Via Networking," www.linkedin.com/pulse/new-survey-reveals-85-all-jobs-filled-via-networking-lou-adler.

5. See NewGradPhysicalTherapy.com, "Leverage Your Volunteering Experience When Applying to Physical Therapy School," newgradphysicaltherapy.com/volunteer-experience-physical-therapy-school.

Chapter 3

1. See the National Center for Education Statistics, "Fast Facts: Graduation Rates," nces.ed.gov/fastfacts/display.asp?id=40.

2. See US Department of Education, "Focusing Higher Education on Student Success," July 27, 2015, www.ed.gov/news/press-releases/fact-sheet-focusing-higher-education-student-success.

3. See TheBalance.com, "Careers in Allied Health Care," February 9, 2018, www.thebalance.com/careers-in-allied-health-care-525853.

4. College Board, "Understanding College Costs," bigfuture.collegeboard.org/pay-for-college/college-costs/understanding-college-costs.

5. See Gap Year Association, "Research Statement," https://www.gapyearassociation.org/research.php.

6. DentalCareersEDU.org, "Becoming a Dental Hygenist," www.dentalcareersedu.org.

7. Virtual Career Network, "Dental Laboratory Technician," www.vcn.org/health-care/careers/51-9081.00/education-training.

8. Federal Student Aid, An Office of the US Department of Education, "FAFSA Changes for 2017–2018," studentaid.ed.gov/sa/about/announcements/fafsa-changes.

Chapter 4

1. Justin Ross Muchnick, *Teens' Guide to College & Career Planning,* 12th ed. (Lawrenceville, NJ: Peterson's, 2015), 179–80.

2. See Mind Tools, "Active Listening: Hear What People Are Really Saying," www.mindtools.com/CommSkll/ActiveListening.htm.

Further Resources

*A*re you looking for more information about the dental health field or even about a branch within a field? Do you want to know more about the college application process or need some help finding the right educational fit for you? Do you want a quick way to search for a good college or school? Try these resources as a starting point on your journey toward finding a great career!

Books

Byers, Ann. *A Career as a Dental Hygienist.* New York: Rosen, 2012.

Field, Shelly. *Career Opportunities in Health Care*, 3rd ed. New York: Checkmark Books, 2007.

Fiske, Edward. *Fiske Guide to Colleges.* Naperville, IL: Sourcebooks, 2018.

Gresham, Barbara B. *Today's Health Professions: Working Together to Provide Quality Care.* Philadelphia: F. A. Davis, 2016.

Henry, Kevin. *Battling and Beating the Demons of Dental Assisting: How Every Dental Assistant Can Have an Amazing, Fulfilling Career.* Oceanside, CA: Indie Books, 2017.

Muchnick, Justin Ross. *Teens' Guide to College & Career Planning*, 12th ed. Lawrenceville, NJ: Peterson's, 2015.

Princeton Review. *The Best 382 Colleges, 2018 Edition: Everything You Need to Make the Right College Choice.* New York: Princeton Review, 2018.

Somervill, Barbara A. *Cool Careers: Dental Hygienist.* Ann Arbor, MI: Cherry Lake, 2010.

Websites

Accrediting Bureau of Health Education Schools
www.abhes.org
This accrediting agency is recognized by the US Department of Education and
by the Council for Higher Education Accreditation. The website includes a list
of accredited institutions and programs, a calendar of upcoming events, a special tab for students, a section on recent publications, and much more.

American Dental Association (ADA)
www.ada.org
The ADA says it's "America's leading advocate for dental health." You'll find
lots of helpful information on their site. From information about careers in
dentistry to special publications to student resources and even a member center
area, this site is a great first stop if you're looking for more information about
all things dental.

American Dental Assistants Association
www.adaausa.org
The ADAA is a professional organization for dental assistants that celebrated
its 93rd year in 2018. The Education tab of this website includes information
about continuing education opportunities, fellowship opportunities, and a page
about CODA-accredited dental assisting programs listed alphabetically by state.

American Dental Hygienists Association
www.adha.org
The ADHA is the largest national organization representing the professional
interests of dental hygienists across the United States. The website includes
information about getting licensed and certified, all about accredited dental hygiene programs, and a student resource center that includes information about
scholarships and grants.

American Gap Year Association
gapyearassociation.org.
The American Gap Year Association's mission is "making transformative gap
years an accessible option for all high school graduates." A gap year is a year

taken between high school and college to travel, teach, work, volunteer, generally mature, and otherwise experience the world. Their website has lots of advice and resources for anyone considering taking a gap year.

The Balance
www.thebalance.com
This site is all about managing money and finances, but also has a large section called Your Career, which provides advice for writing résumés and cover letters, interviewing, and more. Search the site for teens and you can find teen-specific advice and tips.

Commission on Dental Accreditation (CODA)
www.ada.org/en/coda
Part of the ADA, the Commission on Dental Accreditation develops and implements the accreditation standards for dental education programs throughout the United States. Use this site to find CODA-accredited programs and schools near you.

The College Entrance Examination Board
www.collegeboard.org
The College Entrance Examination Board tracks and summarizes financial data from colleges and universities all over the United States. This site can be your one-stop shop for all things college research. It contains lots of advice and information about taking and doing well on the SAT and ACT tests, many articles on college planning, a robust college searching feature, a scholarship searching feature, and a major and career search area. You can type your career of interest (for example, occupational therapy) into the search box and get back a full page that describes the career, gives advice on how to prepare, where to get experience, how to pay for it, what characteristics you should have to excel in this career, lists of helpful classes to take while in high school, and lots of links for more information. A great, well-organized site.

College Grad Career Profile Website
www.collegegrad.com/careers
Although this site is primarily geared toward college graduates, the careers profile area, indicated above, has a list of links to nearly every career you could ever think of. A single click takes you to a very detailed, helpful section that describes the

job in detail, explains the educational requirements, includes links to good colleges that offer this career, includes links to actual open jobs and internships, describes the licensing requirements, if any, lists salaries, and much more.

Commission on Accreditation of Allied Health Education Programs
www.caahep.org
One of the largest programmatic accreditors in the health sciences field. The website enables you to easily search through a large collection of accredited programs. It also includes a specific section just for students and a news and events section.

The DALE Foundation
www.dalefoundation.org
A recognized provider of the American Dental Association, the DALE Foundation maintains information on state requirements that has been compiled by the DANB and state dental boards.

Dental Assisting National Board (DANB)
www.danb.org
The DANB maintains current state information about regional clinical testing requirements on its website and provides links to the appropriate state Boards of Dental Examiners.

Dental Careers EDU
www.dentalcareersedu.org
A great one-stop shop on how to become a dental assistant or dental hygienist. Include links to and information about licensing and certification, how to find a good school, exam information, salary data, and more.

Explore Health Careers Website
www.explorehealthcareers.org
As the title suggests, this site enables you to explore careers in the health fields. You can seek answers to questions such as whether a career in health is right for you or not, find the right fit and focus your search within the many fields, actually find the job or internship you're looking for, learn more about paying for college, and more.

Khan Academy

www.khanacademy.org

The Khan Academy website is an impressive collection of articles, courses, and videos about many educational topics in math, science, and the humanities. You can search any topic or subject (by subject matter and grade), and read lessons, take courses, and watch videos to learn all about it. Includes test prep information for the SAT, ACT, AP, GMAT, and other standardized tests. There is also a College Admissions tab with lots of good articles and information, provided in the approachable Khan style.

Live Career

www.livecareer.com

This site has an impressive number of resources directed toward teens for writing résumés, cover letters, and interviewing.

Mapping Your Future

www.mappingyourfuture.org

This site helps young people figure out what they want to do and maps out how to reach career goals. Includes helpful tips on résumé writing, job hunting, job interviewing, and more.

Monster.com

www.monster.com

Perhaps the most well-known and certainly one of the largest employment websites in the United States. You fill in a couple of search boxes and away you go. You can sort by job title, of course, as well as by company name, location, salary range, experience range, and much more. The site also includes information about career fairs, advice on résumés and interviewing, and more.

National Board for Certification in Dental Laboratory Technology (NBC)

nbccert.org/homepage.cfm

The National Board for Certification in Dental Laboratory Technology (NBC) website lists the current certification requirements to become a CBT (Certified Lab Technician).

Occupational Outlook Handbook
www.bls.gov
The US Bureau of Labor Statistics produces this website. It offers lots of relevant and updated information about various careers, including average salaries, how to work in the industry, the job's outlook in the job market, typical work environments, and what workers do on the job. See www.bls.gov/emp for a full list of employment projections.

Peterson's College Prep
www.petersons.com
In addition to lots of information about preparing for the ACT and SAT tests and easily searchable information about scholarships nationwide, Peterson's site includes a comprehensive searching feature to search for universities and schools based on location, major, name, and more.

Study.com
www.study.com
A site similar to Khan Academy where you can search any topic or subject and read lessons, take courses, and watch videos to learn all about it. Includes a good collection of information about the dental health professions.

TeenLife
www.teenlife.com
This organization calls itself "the leading source for college preparation" and it includes lots of information about summer programs, gap year programs, community service, and more. They believe that spending time out "in the world" outside of the classroom can help students develop important life skills. This site contains lots of links to volunteer and summer programs.

U.S. News & World Report College Rankings
www.usnews.com/best-colleges
U.S. News & World Report provides almost 50 different types of numerical rankings and lists of colleges throughout the United States to help students with their college search. You can search colleges by best reviewed, best value for the money, best liberal arts schools, best schools for B students, and more.

Bibliography

American Dental Association. "Careers in Dentistry." Retrieved July 20, 2018, from www.ada.org/en/education-careers/careers-in-dentistry.

——. "Dental Assistant Job Description." Retrieved July 20, 2018, from www.ada.org/en/education-careers/careers-in-dentistry/dental-team-careers/dental-assistant.

——. "Dental Hygienist Job Description." Retrieved July 20, 2018, from www.ada.org/en/education-careers/careers-in-dentistry/dental-team-careers/dental-hygienist.

——. "Dental Laboratory Technology." Retrieved July 20, 2018, from www.ada.org/en/education-careers/careers-in-dentistry/dental-team-careers/dental-laboratory-technology.

American Dental Education Association (ADEA). "History of Dentistry." Retrieved May 15, 2018, from www.adea.org/GoDental/Health_Professions_Advisors/History_of_Dentistry.aspx.

American Dental Hygienists Association. "Overview Clinical Examinations." Retrieved July 20, 2018, from www.adha.org/resources-docs/7313_Overview_Clinical_Examinations.pdf.

Andrews, Evan. "Did George Washington Have Wooden Teeth?" History.com, April 30, 2014. Retrieved July 10, 2018 from www.history.com/news/did-george-washington-have-wooden-teeth.

TheBalance.com. "Career Choices," February 9, 2018. Retrieved June 10, 2018, from www.thebalance.com/career-choice-or-change-4161891.

Bureau of Labor Statistics, US Department of Labor, Healthcare Occupations website, http://www.bls.gov/ooh/healthcare.

Byers, Ann. *A Career as a Dental Hygienist.* New York: Rosen, 2012.

College Board. "Understanding College Costs." bigfuture.collegeboard.org/pay-for-college/college-costs/understanding-college-costs.

Commission on Dental Accreditation (CODA). "Accreditation." Retrieved July 24, 2018, from www.ada.org/en/coda.

———. "Find a Program." Retrieved July 24, 2018 from www.ada.org/en/coda/accreditation.

DALE Foundation. "How to Earn Your Dental Assistant Certification." Retrieved June 20, 2018, from www.dalefoundation.org/For-Dental-Assistants/How-To-Earn-Your-Dental-Assistant-Certification.

Dental Assisting National Board (DANB). "Become Certified." Retrieved July 19, 2018, from danb.org/Become-Certified.aspx.

DentalCareersEDU.org. "Dental Assistant Requirements for State Licensure and Registration." Retrieved June 16, 2018, from www.dentalcareersedu.org/dental-assistant-requirements-for-state-licensure.

———. "How to Become a Dental Assistant." Retrieved June 16, 2018, from www.dentalcareersedu.org/how-to-become-a-dental-assistant.

———. "Steps to Becoming a Dental Hygienist." Retrieved June 16, 2018, from www.dentalcareersedu.org/how-to-become-a-dental-hygienist.

Field, Shelly. *Career Opportunities in Health Care*, 3rd ed. New York: Checkmark Books, 2007.

Fiske, Edward. *Fiske Guide to Colleges.* Naperville, IL: Sourcebooks, 2018.

Gap Year Association. "Research Statement." Retrieved May 10, 2018, from gapyearassociation.org. https://www.gapyearassociation.org/research.php.

Go College. "Types of Scholarships." Retrieved July 13, 2018, from www.gocollege.com/financial-aid/scholarships/types.

Gresham, Barbara B. *Today's Health Professions: Working Together to Provide Quality Care.* Philadelphia: F. A. Davis, 2016.

Henry, Kevin. *Battling and Beating the Demons of Dental Assisting: How Every Dental Assistant Can Have an Amazing, Fulfilling Career.* Oceanside, CA: Indie Books, 2017.

Isaacs, Kim. "Resume Tips for Healthcare Professionals." Retrieved July 13, 2018, from www.monster.com/career-advice/articlehealthcare-resume-tips.

Joint Commission on National Dental Examinations (JCNDE). "NBDHE General Information." Retrieved June 29, 2018, from www.ada.org/en/jcnde/examinations/national-board-dental-hygiene-examination.

Keates, Cathy. "What Is Job Shadowing?" TalentEgg.ca. Retrieved July 18, 2018, from talentegg.ca/incubator/2011/02/03/what-is-job-shadowing.

LinkedIn.com. "New Survey Reveals 85% of All Jobs Are Filled via Networking." Retrieved July 8, 2018, from www.linkedin.com/pulse/new-survey-reveals-85-all-jobs-filled-via-networking-lou-adler.

Mind Tools. "Active Listening: Hear What People Are Really Saying." Retrieved May 10, 2018, from www.mindtools.com/CommSkll/ActiveListening .htm.

Muchnick, Justin Ross. *Teens' Guide to College & Career Planning*, 12th ed. Lawrenceville, NJ: Peterson's, 2015.

National Board for Certification in Dental Laboratory Technology. "Welcome to NBC." Retrieved July 20, 2018, from https://nbccert.org/homepage .cfm.

National Center for Education Statistics. "Fast Facts: Graduation Rates." Retrieved July 10, 2018, from nces.ed.gov/fastfacts/display.asp?id=40.

Princeton Review. *The Best 382 Colleges, 2018 Edition: Everything You Need to Make the Right College Choice.* New York: Princeton Review, 2018.

Somervill, Barbara A. *Cool Careers: Dental Hygienist.* Ann Arbor, MI: Cherry Lake, 2010.

US Department of Education. "Focusing Higher Education on Student Success," July 27, 2015. Retrieved June 18, 2018, from www.ed.gov/news/ press-releases/fact-sheet-focusing-higher-education-student-success.

Van Buskirk, Peter. "Finding a Good College Fit." *U.S. News & World Report*, June 13, 2011. Retrieved June 18, 2018, from www.usnews .com/education/blogs/the-college-admissions-insider/2011/06/13/finding -a-good-college-fit.

About the Author

Kezia Endsley is an editor and author from Indianapolis, Indiana. In addition to editing technical publications and writing books for teens, she enjoys running and triathlons, traveling, reading, and spending time with her family and seven pets.